Breath
LOVE

Breath
LOVE

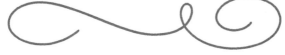

Lauren Chelec Cafritz

Copyright © 2019 by Lauren Chelec Cafritz

ISBN: 978-1-7337955-4-8

Edited by: Tammy Jones and Amy Ashby

Published by Warren Publishing
Charlotte, NC
www.warrenpublishing.net

Printed in the United States

This book is dedicated to my loving parents,
and my amazing husband and sons.

TABLE OF CONTENTS

YOU ARE NOT ALONE

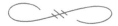

Do you ever feel overwhelmed? Does life seem to bombard you with too much to do and process?

You aren't alone. Every week people come to my practice with similar feelings. And each week, after our breathwork sessions, they leave with a totally different outlook on themselves and their lives.

Breathwork has brought about incredible changes for my clients. I have seen it transform lives—from alleviating chronic body pain and slowing heart rates to boosting immune systems, lifting depression, curbing addictive cravings, and ending toxic drama. Most of all, I have seen it help people open up creatively, manifest their dreams, and make room for love.

These changes—healing and growth—are all within our reach every day, every hour, every minute, every breath. When you learn to connect your breath, you learn to connect to your own power, which is the real magic behind breathwork. I know it sounds too simple, too easy, but it's true. Breathwork gives you a sense of limitless, almost unbridled joy, a feeling of "aliveness." And most amazing of all, this new way of breathing can lead you to a sense of safety, peace, and calm that makes even difficult situations, or challenging jobs and people, something you can handle with grace and ease.

That is what this book is about.

It is about a way of using the power of breath to bring you the confidence, joy, wisdom, creativity, guidance, and peace it has brought me.

Feelings Matter

As a little girl, I was free-spirited, had a ton of energy, and was always in motion. My bounciness and emotions did not fit into my parents' plans. And since both my parents were very young when I was born—and I was their first child— they didn't really know what to do with me. I was a handful. And they were always telling me I was too emotional.

"You're too sensitive!"

No one taught me how to avoid being overwhelmed, so to them, all those big, messy feelings of mine were a problem. My feelings weren't allowed in classrooms, grocery stores, or when trying to fit in with playmates. My feelings were considered disruptive. They needed to be tamped down, ignored, or kept in a box.

"Act your age."

"Get a grip."

"And, no matter what, *no crying*!"

Are these things you were told, or told yourself, growing up?

I can really relate.

My big feelings came with stomachaches. I threw up from anxiety until I was five—sometimes every day. This made me wonder what was wrong with me. I didn't understand my feelings. And I didn't know why I was crying all the time or why I was so angry and upset.

For years I worked on new ways to hide my emotions, in order, I thought, to finally be accepted and loved. Emotions were messy. And I needed to stop making a mess.

So, that's what I did and how I lived. I just stuffed it all in and tamped it all down—that is until I found breathwork. It was then I learned something incredible:

My big feelings are my superpower!

Emotions are what make life worth living. Emotions are real and true, sometimes the only real thing we have; they are what connect us to the present moment and to other people. Emotions make us want to sing. They make us want to dance. They connect us to nature, animals, beauty, and art. They connect us to our aliveness. Our joy. Our juice. Our love.

Emotions are the wellspring of life. *What's more important than emotions?* So how come we hide them, run from them, tamp them down, or numb them?

Big Feelings Are a Gift

Here's the reality: Big feelings and emotions are a gift. They give us energy, passion, and power. Since most of us haven't been raised to accept and embrace them, they scare us. We are afraid to feel them. They make us feel out of control. We haven't learned how to harness their *power*. We haven't learned to do that by harnessing the power of our breath—yet.

Harness the power of breath?

3

Yep, you heard me right. Breath is the key to being able to be with our feelings instead of stashing them away in a box under the bed. And by experiencing our breath, we can learn to unleash our own power, energy, creativity, and passion. Breath is where our magic is, where our spirit resides.

Breathwork strengthens our understanding of our feelings and allows us to experience them, accept them, and integrate them so they work for us and not against us.

Feelings don't have to be scary or knock us off balance. Events in life that cause big feelings to arise—a breakup, an illness, a job change—become more manageable and less stressful once you learn how to breathe with them. Breathwork teaches us how to relax and let go of fear. You learn to ride the waves of your feelings rather than be wiped out by them. You learn how to embrace and trust your feelings, and then you are on your way to harnessing their power.

Your energy will change. And your life will change too. You'll become more resilient, more authentic, more creative, more juicy, more loving, and more whole. Get ready to laugh louder, cry harder, and feel more alive!

Change your breath.
Change your mind.
Change your life.

My Intention for This Book

Each breathwork session begins by creating or setting an intention. Setting an intention is important in any endeavor. Our intentions allow us to become crystal clear about our hopes and goals. They're a way of sending ourselves an important message, so our subconscious and conscious selves are aligned in a mission.

Setting an intention works something like this—say you've decided you want to swim to an island in the distance. The island gives you a point of reference, a place where you want to land. That island is your *intention*. By saying your intention out loud, you help manifest it into being. Before you know it, almost by magic, you are standing on the shore of that island. We all have the power to manifest our goals. Believe me, this works!

I find great joy in helping people use breathwork to find the strength and energy to move forward. Whether it's leaping into a career change, starting a relationship or ending one, riding through a health challenge, or creating positive life changes, people discover a new way of being and living through breathwork.

So, here's my intention for *Breath LOVE*: To help deepen your connection to your breath and yourself, to enhance your life in big beautiful ways, to encourage you to be brave and ride the waves of your emotions with a smile. To empower you on your own breath journey.

Let's get started!

CHAPTER 1

BREATH IS MAGIC

Breath is everything. It gives us life.

It fuels all of our movements and actions. It allows our lungs to expand, our hearts to pump blood, and our brains to throttle ahead. When was the last time you thought about how you are breathing? Unless you are running a marathon, sitting in a yoga class, having an asthma attack, or giving birth, the chances are you haven't. Even then, you may not have given *all of your attention* to the depth of your inhale and the release of your exhale. You were probably focused on a difficult yoga pose—or dealing with the pain of pushing a baby out of what seemed like way too small a hole.

Most people first encounter "conscious breathing" while taking a yoga or childbirth class. Breathwork uses various breathing techniques—taught in individual or group settings—to promote self-awareness and enhancement of physical, emotional, cognitive, and spiritual wellbeing. Breathing can get us through a lot. There's much more to know, though, and much more to savor from every single breath you take.

Each inhalation, each exhalation, can be a pathway to joy, to love, to living a full and authentic life. Each breath links us directly to our minds, our hearts, and our souls.

There is no such thing as an unimportant breath.

Don't Look Up!

None of this occurred to me either, until I had a problem. Breathwork lessons? *You've got to be joking.* I didn't have a woo-woo bone in my body (that I knew of) in those days. I was a photojournalist, taking a little maternity break after having my first baby. He was a restless and colicky little guy. My husband and I were getting no sleep.

Confession: I approached motherhood the way I approached everything else I did in those days—total perfection was mandatory. I was high-strung, something of an overachiever, and I took pride in being able to make things happen in the real world. The idea of a "spiritual awakening" was totally foreign to me, and I didn't ever expect to have one.

Spirituality wasn't my thing. Anxiety *was*. My husband used to say that any little thing could launch me into a code-red state of alarm. Like, if I had a cough and a fever, I must have the flu. If I got into a fight with a friend, it must be signaling the end of the friendship. Scary things were always around the corner.

My mind was full of fear.

Wasn't everybody's?

I thought code-red was normal.

Our son was about nine months old when my neck started to really bother me. It was painful to carry my baby around. The pain was so bad, I couldn't turn my neck.

I'm not talking about an ache or stiffness. I'm talking an insane, burning-nerve kind of pain, like sciatica in my neck. It felt like a live wire in the back of my head was attached to a sparking jumper cable. Before long, I was code-red 24/7, just trying to deal with the pain. And I was desperate to figure out how to make it go away. When I got a body massage, I was told my neck and shoulders were really tight, so I booked more massages. When the pain was still there, I saw spine specialists who told me I would need surgery in the near future.

My grandfather was a doctor, a general practitioner, whom everybody in my family loved and revered. So, we've always taken our faith in Western medicine personally. Whatever a medical expert told me, I believed.

"This doesn't look good," the neurosurgeon told me.

"What should I do?" I asked.

"Just don't look up."

I thanked him and, following this advice, I barely ever looked up for the next six years. My neck pain never really went away. No matter what I did, I thought about my neck first, and I babied it. There was no way I was getting that surgery.

And it's not that I didn't try other fixes. As anybody with chronic pain will tell you, there are lots of fixes, or supposed fixes, and lots of different avenues to explore and work your way through. I went to different massage therapists, physiatrists (a doctor who works with the muscles around an injured area), and physical therapists. I was told to strengthen my neck and also try gentle yoga, which uses chairs and blocks and pillows—all kinds of props—because everybody in the class had some type of injury or limitation.

Gentle yoga helped. It really did. I could move my neck more, and that made me hopeful and excited. So, I signed up for more classes.

The Ultimate Rush

Then something happened in gentle yoga one day. I was doing a pose and felt a huge current of energy rocket through me. It was a throbbing energy, really powerful.

Nothing gentle about it.

My heart beat and boomed in my chest.

Just when I caught my breath, another surge of energy came. I was sweating by then and frantic. The strange sensation was so intense, I wondered if I was having a heart attack. I didn't know whether to relax with it or go to the hospital. On the verge of panic, I asked the yoga instructor to help me.

Did she know what was happening?

She didn't.

That made me flip out even more.

As soon as I got home, I called my GP—and went into her office immediately. She gave me a prescription for Valium.

An "anxiety attack." That's what she said it was.

I was anxious and just needed a tranquilizer to calm me down.

Except, I kept having these "attacks" and the more I had, the worse they got. The currents of feeling became more powerful, and scarier. My heart would start palpitating and I would become short of breath. I felt so helpless and out of control. My fear only compounded the problem. I felt like I needed more Valium. At first I was taking one quarter of a pill, then ramped it up to one half. Finally, I needed a whole pill to calm me down. This made only a small dent. The surging current would go away for ten minutes, but come roaring back. Knowing I was getting worse, I saw the doctor again and learned that my anxiety attacks were now more like panic attacks. And I never knew when they would come. That made everything worse. I couldn't do anything without worrying an attack would come. Even my gentle yoga classes felt like walking through a field of landmines. The "attacks" were taking over my life. I couldn't even drive anymore.

A good friend of mine, a musician I've known my whole life, offered to take me to see a breathworker who he went to and liked.

Connected Breath

The breathworker was soothing and talked to me for a while, then asked me to lie down on a mattress on the floor of her quiet, peaceful breathwork room. My breath was shallow—tight short inhalations, stammering exhalations. Stressed out, fight-or-flight, survival-mode breathing.

Then the breathworker asked me to breathe with her, following her deeper, slower rhythmic patterns, and explained how to "connect" my breath. She asked me to connect my inhale to my exhale and right back to my inhale, watching to see that there was no space between each.

As soon as my breath was connected, I felt a strange energy coming through me—sensations I wasn't used to, like tingling and twitching. It was as if certain parts of my body were seizing up more, holding onto tension. I felt one of my anxiety waves starting. A super-powerful one.

I froze.

"Here comes a strong wave!" I warned the breathworker, still bracing myself. She put her hand on my arm, very softly. Her voice was low and calm.

"Why don't you just stay with it," she said, "and describe it to me?"

"It's a strong sensation, a huge energy wave," I answered, my voice getting tighter. "A throbbing wave. I feel so afraid. I can feel it in my chest."

My sense of fear was intense. I was on the edge of panic.

"Lauren, that's energy," she said. "That's you. You're afraid of you—*your own power.*"

This took me a second to process.

"That's me? *My own power?*"

"That's you."

It took another moment for this to sink in. And by then, my heart palpitations had stopped. I kept trying to follow the flow of my breath and gradually felt calmer, so much calmer. Later, she explained that the first "attack" in the yoga class had been a pretty routine energy rush that comes when we release stuck energy—something they never told me about in yoga, but which isn't uncommon. Not knowing anything about it, my own fear escalated the sensation and drove me into full-blown panic.

The breathworker explained to me that emotion is just energy in motion. When our energy is stuck, she said, it hurts. By getting energy "unstuck," by moving or breathing, the tightness and constriction eased and the energy could flow.

She introduced another concept that sent my mind reeling. At the end of the day, she said, all our feelings can be boiled down to love and fear. This seemed overly simplistic to me at first. There were so many different emotions inside me. *How could everything boil down to only two feelings?*

Love or fear?

The more I thought about this, the more true it seemed. When we are afraid and feel out of control, we go into resistance mode, or "fear" mode, to protect ourselves. If we are feeling more balanced and strong, we are able to do the opposite—accept and embrace things coming our way.

Each breath session was easier. The breathworker was always soothing and calm, her breathwork space safe and comforting. I learned to ride the waves of energy that showed up as different sensations in the body. I learned to breathe, let go, and reconnect with myself—try to accept my big emotions and listen to my smaller, quieter ones. Before long, I felt more in control and also more alive, more in love with life, and more creative.

On top of that, the pain in my neck slowly went away.
How did that happen?

Looser and Happier

It's probably not a big surprise that being a new mother had something to do with my neck pain. With the help of breathwork, I was able to figure out that some of my relationships—important ones—were not in alignment after my transition to motherhood.

Everything in a marriage changes with a baby, and it requires a whole new conversation and level of honesty. Parenthood also causes changes in your relationships with friends, your work, and your own parents. You suddenly have insights into your relationship with your mom and dad that maybe you didn't even bother thinking about before.

What happened to me is really common. I was suffering the way a lot of new mothers suffer—overwhelmed by changes in every aspect of my life. Transitions are hard for many of us. Gratefully, breathwork gave me a safe place and safe way to reevaluate my relationships. It empowered me to make changes, and more conscious ones.

And breathwork led me to something I never expected: a spiritual awakening. When you give yourself a chance to be authentically you and connect to your breath, there's a spiritual element to it. When that happens, you become more aligned with your spiritual self. That alone gives you a feeling of calm, confidence, and centeredness.

I started seeing things differently after just a few sessions. I felt safer. I felt calmer. I felt a sense of faith and trust in life, in God or Spirit, or whatever you want to call the force that runs through all of us and all living things.

That connection is a lovely feeling.

I felt taken care of.

I felt loved.

And eventually I calmed down about motherhood. Wow, that was a relief. I could find more humor and be less neurotic. My husband saw it right away. And over time, especially after our second son was born, the difference breathwork made in my life became profound. Parenting is freaking hard! It's always testing your limits. The minute you think you've got it down, your kids enter a whole new phase and everything changes again. Breathwork, even in my first few sessions, helped me get comfortable with change. My own changes—and everyone else's too.

Along with calm, confidence, and centeredness came a feeling of softness. Before I started breathing, I was just a tight ball. Not just my neck was tight, but my entire body and being were tight. That's what perfectionism does to us. I was stressed out and nervous about doing things right all the time. And I had been trying to "make" my boys perfect too—no fighting, no throwing balls in the house. "Get your homework done!"

I knew I had changed, but didn't know how much until my younger son's camp counselors reported one summer that he wore the same shirt for an entire month and I just laughed. *Like, so what*? So, I've got the messy, rebellious kid. Oh well. Big deal. Right?

Each year brought more confidence and calm. The more work I did on myself, and the more conscious breaths I took, the more I was able to master not just my breath, but my emotions too. The concepts I had learned in my early breathwork sessions became clearer and clearer to me. Feelings really did boil down to love and fear. I wanted to choose love. I wanted to share love, bathe in love, and let love flow through me to others. Rather than tight and shutdown, I wanted to feel loose and happy. I wanted to feel responsive, present, open, and soft. And the more breathwork I did, the more I wanted to do. The feeling of being connected to myself and capable of handling whatever sensations came my way was *empowering*.

I wanted to learn more, feel more, and understand more about breathwork, like *how on earth did it work*?

Look Down at Your Ruby Slippers

Now I am a breathwork teacher and facilitator, certified by two different schools of breathwork, who has done years of coaching in my own private breathwork practice. Each year of teaching and working with private clients has only deepened my convictions about the benefits of breathwork.

And when people I meet ask me how something as simple as an involuntary body function can be so powerful, I say it's a little like Dorothy and her ruby slippers in *The Wizard of Oz*. All Dorothy wants is to get back home to Kansas. And she thinks she needs to see the wizard so he can perform some kind of magic to get her there again. She walks and walks along the yellow brick road, encountering danger and conflicts and, well, you know how it ends.

All she had to do was click her heels together.

She was wearing her ruby slippers the whole time!

It's the same with breath. We always have it—a pathway to a better life, a pathway home—but we haven't really been taught to use it. In the end, it is not the slippers that save Dorothy. She awakens to the power she's had inside her all along. Awareness is key. Awareness is all it takes.

The answer isn't me. I am not a wizard. I'm more like Glinda, the good witch, who tells Dorothy to just look down at her shoes.

The answer is in *you*.

My job is to help you look inside and connect with a power that's always been with you.

Now, let's try something. Take five deep breaths, connecting your inhale to your exhale, a seamless flow of air coming into you, and going out, with no space between each breath.

Try and create slow, steady calm breaths.

Feel the floor under your feet.

Feel the back of the chair supporting you.

With every inhale, feel the expansion inside you. With every exhale just relax, taking a moment to reconnect to that power that's been in you all along.

Let's keep going.

The
answer
is in
you.

CHAPTER 2

FEELING COZY, COMFY, AND SAFE

I was once skiing and, after dropping onto a steep run, I turned a corner and directly in front of me, right on my path, a woman was on the ground writhing in pain. She had wiped out and hurt herself really badly. She was in distress and could barely talk.

While my husband went for help, I crouched next to her. "I teach people how to breathe," I said. "May I help you?" She nodded and I put my hand on her belly.

"Focus on my hand," I said. "Breathe into my hand."

Without saying a word, she started breathing into my hand. I could feel her belly moving under her bulky ski suit. By the time she had taken seven deep breaths, her face had relaxed. By the time the medics came, she was able to joke and laugh. Her own breath had worked faster than any drug. It was like a superhighway that took her away from fear and pain to a place of calm and peace.

Breath took her to a place where she felt safe.

are more fearful than others. That's just how
If you have been told, like I was, that you
sitive" and "too emotional," there's a good
chance you feel more anxious and fearful too. You've
probably got a big imagination and it is really good at
dreaming up all kinds of awful stuff to be scared about. If
your imagination keeps that up, it can become a habit. You
can find yourself in a chronic state of dread, always worried
what surprises tomorrow will bring.

We all have normal stresses to cope with; we're holding
down a job, raising our kids, staying out of danger, staying
out of trouble. Life has lots of moving parts, and lots of
unknowns. Additional stress can pile on if our environment
is turbulent and unpredictable, or if the world around us
feels off-kilter and is changing too fast. We like things to be
stable and more predictable.

Many people are feeling edgy and irritable these days,
their minds whirling with worries. Lots of people feel out of
control. Stuff comes up fast—too many negative surprises!
Life for many people has become an icy downhill run that's
scary to navigate. New clients who come to my breathwork
practice remind me of the woman I met on the ski slope.
They've wiped out and are writhing in distress.

The more out of control we feel, the more afraid we are.

Fear is so chronic and pervasive in modern life, we
barely notice it anymore.

But we know we feel something …

We feel tight.

We feel anxious.

We can't sleep.

You can see fear in the stressed-out way people drive
and honk at each other. You can see it in the way they talk
and what they talk about—sharing negative outcomes. You

can see it in their posture and on their faces, the worry and frown lines.

You can see it in how they breathe.

An anxious person takes tight shallow breaths. Shallow chest breathing means you are in "fight-or-flight" mode—the kind of breathing soldiers in combat have, or anybody facing physical danger. I was a shallow chest breather when I went for my first breathwork session.

What do I mean by shallow?

A shallow breath happens up in our chest and the belly does not move. The breath is tight and constricted, and it could be choppy and uneven. Put two hands on your belly and take a deep breath into your hands. Notice if your hands move out on your inhale. If they do, shift one hand to your chest and practice breathing from your belly up to your chest. This is called a diaphragmatic breath.

If your hands do not move on your belly as you inhale, then keep them both there and continue focusing on breathing into your belly and getting your hands to rise as you take a deep breath. If your belly still does not move, no worries, keep reading. There are many reasons for this, and it's part of your journey. Everybody takes a shallow breath from time to time. It's a part of the natural response to being startled—when cortisol and adrenaline are released into our bloodstream. Shallow breathing only becomes a problem when it becomes a habit. If you have lived with fear or anxiety for a long time, or experienced trauma, your breath can get stuck in this fight-or-flight mode, even after the danger and pain have long passed. You haven't moved on from fight-or-flight because you are still afraid or you haven't let go of something. You've stuffed your emotions deep inside.

Until I tried breathwork, I had probably been gasping along in fear-mode my whole life. I had no idea there was another way to breathe. It didn't take more than a few sessions before I was beginning to feel very different.

Almost as if my entire way of approaching the world and my life had altered. I felt calmer and more centered. It was hard to believe. *Just by breathing differently?*

It was simple, shockingly simple. By breathing in a conscious and connected way, I was sending a message to my entire being—my mind, my body, and my soul: I was safe.

Feeling safe is the beginning of healing.

Valium couldn't do that.

But my breath could.

The Breathwork Cocoon

Most clients come to see me for the first time because they are afraid of something.

"I'm scared of having a baby."

"My son is leaving home for college."

"I'm unhappy in my relationship and I don't know what to do."

At first they just want to cope. They have heart palpitations and want them to stop. And they'd really like to be able to sleep through the night, or stop losing it when their kids do something to upset them.

Sometimes they have no idea what they are anxious about. They are experiencing a free-floating kind of unidentified anxiety. They tell me they are having "panic attacks"—similar to what I had. Their doctors have referred them to me because medications or talk therapy alone have not helped them.

Bottom line?

It seems like life is throwing them a curveball. Things are changing up too quickly. They are living with lots of transitions and uncertainty—the stuff that really strikes fear in most people.

They don't feel safe.

And when people don't feel safe, they can't breathe.

That's why a soothing environment is such an important part of doing breathwork, the same way it is for massage therapy. Whether I am working with a group in a large studio or giving a private session in my own breathwork room, I create a calm space in which clients feel comfortable and relaxed. I keep the lighting low and often use candles. I keep lots of pillows, bolsters, and blankets nearby so clients are warm and comfortable.

There are lots of studies about this—how people heal faster and do better with pain, recovery, and fear of the unknown in an environment that feels safe and welcoming. I am always making improvements to my breathwork space, making it cozier and quieter. I like to think of it as a cocoon where transformational magic can happen.

If you are doing breathwork at home, or any kind of meditation, the same thing applies. Find a warm and quiet place where you can't be interrupted—away from the phone, computer, or doorbell.

Manifesting Mojo

In my group classes, we sit in a circle at the start of the breathwork session and begin by taking twenty connected breaths together. This changes the feeling in the room almost immediately, because breathing in this way takes us into a different part of our brains or minds. It carries us out of the amygdala, or primitive brain, and gets us into the prefrontal cortex, which is the creative, higher reasoning part of the brain.

Taking just seven deep breaths can make that happen. Twenty breaths … even better.

The way we breathe affects our blood chemistry. A diaphragmatic breath sends a signal to our central nervous system that we're not under threat. There's no danger. We're okay. As soon as that happens, the cortisol and adrenaline levels in our bloodstream—the chemicals that keep us buzzing and on edge—begin to drop. It feels like we've entered a totally different state of mind, a more relaxed and quiet one.

We might do some warm-up movements, raising our arms up with an inhale and down with a noisy exhale. It's not unlike some warm-ups in yoga.

Then we come to a really important part of every session: setting intention. Words are powerful. What we say to ourselves, we make happen. Positive intentions can help us get unstuck. We go around our circle, person by person. We keep things simple. We keep things short. We make declarative statements in the present tense. For instance, if you're having tons of anxiety, you declare that you are already calm.

You say, "I am calm."

Or, "I am peaceful and calm."

Simple is more powerful, right? There's no need to get overly specific and wordy about it. Intentions are best if they are pure, direct, and straightforward. Let's say you are feeling low energy. A lot of my clients in the city are chronically tired and feel overwhelmed. Your intention might be: "I am energetic and calm."

Tired could mean stuck, and sometimes it could mean you're feeling down. So, you might want to say, "I am open and flowing." Or "I am flowing and joyful."

Or maybe you're feeling cold. Lots of people feel a body temperature shift when they are anxious. So, your intention might be: "I am warm and safe."

Some people are saddened by gloomy weather. When it rains for days on end, they feel grey and sad: "I am sunny and playful."

wise

loving

creative

calm

flowing   joyful

peaceful   *I am*

warm   safe

enough

confident

powerful

Or let's say you are having a hard time finding a job. You keep going to interviews and being turned down: "I am enough."

Entire books have been written on this alone. Setting an intention is how we come to manifest amazing things in our lives. It's how we get the things we want and need, and how we nourish ourselves. You say an intention and it begins to grow and grow and grow. Your intention is where you want to be. *How you want to feel.* Your intention directs your spirit and tells it what to create.

Let's try it out. Take a moment to check in with yourself and see where you are, how you're feeling, and what you wish you had more of in your life. Then put the words "I am" in front of that word that describes how you'd like to feel. *I am joyful. I am vibrant.*

Now say that out loud—or, if you aren't in a place where you feel comfortable doing that, just say it silently in your mind while you begin to breathe. Keep breathing for ten breaths and keep allowing that intention to play in your mind and begin to imagine owning that intention fully.

Practice this every day until the intention becomes your way of being. To help you along, you could also add some sounds and tastes and other sensory details to your intention. These can make them more tangible, more real to you. Once, after suggesting this to a client in a breathwork session, she came up with a new intention for herself.

"I am peaceful," she said.

"How does that smell?" I asked.

"It smells like ocean air."

"How does it taste?" I asked.

"It tastes fresh."

"And how does it feel?"

"Smooth."

Peaceful, ocean air, fresh, and smooth.

Who wouldn't want to experience that?

Pushing Pleasure

A woman appeared in my group class one week. She was from South America, about thirty years old, and early in her pregnancy, just four months along. You could barely tell. When the class formed a circle at the beginning of class, she explained that she wanted to learn how to breathe so she wouldn't feel so anxious about childbirth.

Her mother and her mother's mother had really painful birth experiences, she said, and had scared her with awful stories. Childbirth was five months away and she was already heading toward full-blown panic. "I don't want to be panicked," she said. "I want to be excited in the birthing room. I want to feel joy."

I love it when a pregnant woman comes to me with a big beautiful intention like that. Instead of saying, "*I need to get through this,*" the woman was actually asking for more—for a peak experience in life. This woman didn't just want to cope; she wanted to be filled with joy while having her baby.

We talked about what she wanted her experience to feel like. I suggested she keep coming to class and explained how her childbirth could be different than the stories she heard from her mother and grandmother.

She mustered a smile. Underneath it, I could see she was very tight and constricted. And her breath was shallow. She was barely breathing at all. It was the opposite of where she wanted to wind up.

Any birth doula or midwife will tell you the same thing: The looser your mind feels while giving birth, the looser your body will be. We are healthiest, and most vibrant, when we're open and flowing. The minute we're tight and anxious, that just hurts the whole process—any process. A big part of childbirth is learning how to relax with discomfort, whether it's mental or physical.

How loose could you possibly feel while giving birth?

So loose you could French kiss somebody you love! I'm not kidding. The pregnancy gurus advise the same thing for an easier birth. Loosen those lips and relax your jaw! If your mouth is tight, your cervix will be too.

I was happy to see the pregnant woman show up in class again the following week. She didn't seem any looser or more relaxed, though. If anything, she seemed tighter. She did the opening class exercises, created an intention, and tried to open her breath, but it was still shallow and tight. She rarely laughed or showed much emotion. The next week, the same thing. If she felt a new sensation, like when the baby began wiggling around inside her, she would tense up with fearful thoughts. *Oh, it's going to be painful!*

My role as a breathworker was to help her figure out how to get to a place where she could feel okay with sensations, both comfortable and uncomfortable. Once she could breathe with those sensations in a breath session, it would become easier to do that during delivery.

Week after week, she kept coming. It was interesting to watch the layers fall off. It wasn't until her seventh month of pregnancy—after about 12 classes—that she was able to truly loosen up. Her breathing became open and flowing. She had a luxuriant inhale and a big, open, relaxed exhale.

She told the class a bit more about her life. She seemed lonely. She was far away from her parents and family in South America. Her husband traveled for work a lot.

That month, she began laughing in class. She felt safe to cry. And as she became more comfortable with being open, being vulnerable, she started moving her hips and yawning big yawns to open up her jaws and mouth. She was slowly letting go of fear, facing and letting go of past wounds and stories. Each week, there were new things for her to face and discover. It turned out she had been bullied pretty severely as a young girl, and she let go of that. Other fears, old stories, old programming appeared in her pathway that had affected her breath patterns.

She kept breathing.

She let go.

She moved on—feeling lighter and stronger.

Not everybody who comes to breathwork is so committed. All her effort was paying off. At eight months, she was blossoming. We put more pillows around her, asked her about baby names, and if she'd gotten a crib yet. To be more comfortable, she was doing all her breathwork on her side, instead of being propped up.

One week, she didn't come to class.

We were all asking each other, "Anyone seen her? What's going on?"

Not long afterward, she sent the most beautiful photo of herself holding her baby girl right after the birth. In the photograph, her smile radiated complete love and happiness.

It was the biggest smile you've ever seen.

All the things she'd learned in class showed up in her birthing process, she told me later. When she got contractions, she didn't give into fear. She relaxed with them, and breathed with them. She trusted her breath, and just stayed with her breath. It was like being with a trusted old friend. Her breath gave her comfort, security, a feeling of calm. Instead of reliving the stories her mom had told her—that she was a "painful" birth—she was able to welcome her own daughter with excitement and joy. She said it was the most powerful experience of her life.

Her baby wasn't a pain but a huge blessing.

And so was she. She became empowered. She realized she wasn't her mother and her grandmother. What had happened to them didn't need to happen to her. It was safe for her to be her own person, to have her own authenticity. She had come for help with the birthing process and wound up learning to accept and love herself along the way.

That Safe Space Inside You

When you face something really huge and looming that you were once terribly afraid of—childbirth, sadness, a bad memory, a scary story you were told when you were little—and continue conscious connected breathing, something happens. You have created a home for yourself inside you, a refuge, a place that is beyond pain and fear.

Where you are strong.

Where you are joyful.

Where you are safe.

You begin to feel how powerful you are. Your spirit can take on a lot. And rather than tamping down your energy and emotion into a small box, you can learn to use it. People often come to breathwork for one thing and stay to heal other things. They see that they have more work to do—and more to gain. Feeling empowered is addictive. Living in fear starts to seem like a choice. And a choice you don't want.

Sounds too simple, right? *All this from a natural reflex?* Remember that icy downhill run where I encountered the injured woman writhing in pain and distress on the ground? How many breaths did it take before her face totally changed and her body loosened?

Seven.

Now I'd like you to take seven deep, connected, cozy breaths to see what that magic number—seven—can do for you, right now.

On every inhale, breathe in the sensation of feeling fully safe. On the exhale, melt into the coziness of a soft blanket and the feeling of a warm hug. Keep connecting your inhale and exhale seamlessly. Notice any sensations you may feel after only seven breaths. If you're ready to dive in deeper and hang out longer, go further. Try twenty breaths.

And when you can, keep reading.

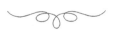

Feeling
empowered
is
addictive.

CHAPTER 3

THE NOISY SIGH (OR, HOW TO RELEASE YOUR INNER CRITIC WITH LOVE)

Think back to when you were five years old. Were you full of energy, always bouncing around and excited about life? Were you quietly playing in the dirt, studying bugs?

Were you criticized for what you did? Were you teased? Were your feelings hurt? Did you feel bad about yourself?

Even if you weren't as super-sensitive and high-strung as I was as a child, you can probably relate to what I'm saying. When we are little, the big people in our lives are always telling us what we need to fix about ourselves in order to fit in.

It hurts to be criticized.

It hurts to be teased, or not liked.

It's painful to feel like you aren't enough.

So, in order to fit in, we try to change who we are. We shut pieces of ourselves down. To keep getting praise for behaving ourselves—the praise and love we feel we need—we become our own critics. We are always minding ourselves and criticizing ourselves.

Here's the worst part: At some point on the road to adulthood, the critic inside us takes over. That joyful and exuberant child inside is always kept tamped down, silent. That child spends their whole life barely breathing, squeezed into shoes that are too tight.

You can reverse this! You can connect to your unbridled joy, your childish wonder, your authentic spark. You can let the bright and sparkly part of you out to play and create. That child is still inside you.

That's the secret I learned during my early breathwork sessions. When I learned to breathe, a full inhale connected to a fully relaxed exhale, I was able to say goodbye to the grouchy tough critic inside me most of the time. I was able to let go of the voice inside my head that told me I didn't measure up to my parents' expectations. That's the voice that had been keeping me in fear mode and making me feel tight and constricted.

This chapter is about self-judgment and how it keeps all of us living in fear, tightness, pain, and anxiety. It's about how breathing can help you release your inner critic and release your feelings of self-doubt. Breathing can shift you out of fear mode and allow you to live with heart and courage. The process is simple. I've seen it work countless times.

Sometimes it only takes a breath. How is that possible? Because all emotions are just energy—or energy in motion. It's really that basic. The way to say goodbye to your inner critic is to connect to your breath and create an intention.

Try this one: *I am enough.*

Seem too simple? Let's practice doing a big noisy sigh. I think you'll see what I mean. Take three full breaths in through the nose and out through the mouth.

On the exhale, try making some noise. You can do it! Let out a noisy sigh on the exhale and with every exhale after that, see how much more you can release.

Each exhale is a chance to let go, and keep letting go of the stories that leave you feeling not enough.

Life becomes easier and a lot more fun. Mistakes aren't so uncomfortable. Transitions become manageable.

Energy is just energy.

It comes. It goes.

Let the bright and sparkly part of you out to play.

Breathing Hot and Wiry

A soccer player came to see me a few years ago. He was a young high school student and college recruit, a massively talented athlete with everything going for him. Speed. Strength. Quick reflexes. Physical and spatial intelligence. He seemed to have it all together.

Except for one thing: his emotions.

He kept getting super angry while playing, especially when the stakes were high. Under stress, he'd lose it during a match or just freeze.

This kind of red-hot anger can be debilitating. Some people's anger just gets so intense and dramatic, they become wrapped up in it, and almost addicted to the drama and the story of the anger, until it becomes this snarly ball of hot lava.

What was behind the soccer star's rage?

He was very critical of himself. If he made a mistake or had trouble getting the ball back, he became consumed with self-judgment. His fear of failure and feeling of being unworthy took the form of anger. And that emotion only compounded the problem. He'd get so angry with himself, his concentration would crash and his playing would go down the tubes.

In our first breathwork session, after we'd worked on connecting his breath, I wanted to help him see that emotion is just energy. He didn't need to put a label on his feelings. He didn't need to tell himself lots of stories about it. And he didn't need to beat himself up for losing his temper. Rather than telling me about how angry he was, I asked him to recall what that energy felt like when he lost the ball.

"It feels hot," he said. "And it feels wiry."

I asked him to take a minute and visualize that he had lost the ball in a game—and the hot and wiry sensation was coming up.

We were breathing together, conscious connected breaths, and it only took a minute for him to nod. He was ready.

"Do you have the hot and wiry feeling?"

"Yes."

"Okay, so can you breathe with it?"

He nodded again. In his mind, he began breathing into the hot and wiry feeling, breathing along with it, as if joining the feeling with his breath.

"It is just energy, right?" I said. "No need to think of it any other way. There's no story. There's no word except energy. Just breathe with it."

"Okay," he said. After a breath or two, he let out a really noisy sigh. It was long and loud and husky. The body releases energy and emotion in different ways. His noisy sigh meant he had released some energy—and let go of stories, labels, probably a bunch of self-judgment. His entire body seemed lighter, easier.

He was looser and relaxed.

"What's happening?" I asked.

"It's gone," he said, smiling, and a little puzzled.

It only took an hour or two for him to absorb the basic lesson of emotions and energy. The next time he froze during a match—he was playing in Brazil and lost the ball in a crucial moment of the game—he began breathing into the hot and wiry sensation when it came up. And he used that energy to get the ball back again.

I saw him only one more time after that. He got it. Energy is only energy.

Our stories and words can keep us stuck.

Our overthinking keeps us stuck.

And by breathing into the hot and wiry sensation and not attaching a story to it, the energy he had been experiencing came and went.

Energy comes. Energy goes.

He released it with a beautiful, noisy sigh.

Using Your Energy (or E-Motion)

Emotion is energy in motion. I'll probably say that another one hundred times in this book. *Let it sink in!* There's no need to make it more complicated than that. Lots of times when people say they are troubled by their feelings, or afraid of them, they are just afraid of feeling their own energy.

Breathwork drives this reality home. Once you are able to see for yourself, the way the soccer player did, that emotions are just energy in motion, you can release them and move on with your life rather than attaching yourself to lots of cumbersome stories. And once you get some distance on it, and see the energy as just energy—and not personal—you can choose to use it for things that are more creative, healthier, and more life-affirming.

Emotions can leave us feeling out of control.

Energy is something we can harness.

E-motion is Energy in Motion

I have another story about this. A woman in her thirties came to see me. She had a demanding job and set high standards for herself. Like the soccer player, she carried around lots of self-judgment stories in her head. This became a problem for her at work. Every time she was in a meeting and had to speak up and explain something she was doing, or defend a decision she'd made, her face began to flush. It was like a hot flash, except she was too young for menopause. And it was definitely triggered by emotions. It always went with a feeling she labeled as "panic" and "anxiety."

If these "flushes" weren't so noticeable to everybody else in the office, I'm not sure she would have come to see me. In her mind, she had an embarrassing problem she wanted to make go away.

After we'd done some connected breathing together, I asked her to visualize the last time she'd had a "flush" in a meeting. What happened to get her feeling panicky?

She said she had been feeling under the gun, on the defense. She was disappointed in herself and worried she was not up to her job. She felt like a fraud. Sitting in a meeting, she had felt enormous pressure to perform and at the same time, she felt she was letting herself down.

The stories in her head were ones you might be familiar with, because so many of us spend our waking hours in a self-defeating, trash-talking conversation with ourselves:

"I'm not smart enough."

"I'm not good at this."

"I'm not up to this job."

"I'm not worthy."

My client whose face flushed in work meetings wasn't really experiencing the moment, or even truly present at the meeting. In her head, she heard only the voice of her inner critic that was connected to all the other tall tales she carried around with her—a.k.a. "*baggage.*" It took her back to the other times in her life when she felt she'd let somebody down or wasn't good enough.

In our first session together, as soon as she realized she was being triggered, the first big lesson was learning how to say goodbye to all those "I'm-not-worthy" stories. Lots of us have those tales kicking around our heads. But why allow them to stay there? For most of us, though, these stories have been around so long we're used to them.

You can learn how to calm those stories down, quiet them to a whisper until they don't cause the same reactions anymore. That way, you won't feel triggered or become unhinged by them. Once they are quieter, you can start learning to ride the waves of those feelings like a pro-surfer.

I asked the woman to describe how it felt when her face flushed.

"Is it comfortable or uncomfortable energy?"

"Uncomfortable," she said.

Then I asked how the uncomfortable energy felt. Was it sluggish and heavy? Or maybe fast and jarring? Hot or cold or tight?

She thought for a second.

"Hot and jumpy."

I asked if she could close her eyes and relive a moment in a meeting when she felt the sensation of feeling hot and jumpy.

Yes, she could. And she closed her eyes. A few moments later, she nodded. She was ready.

When she felt that hot rush coming, and the jumpy energy rising in her body, I told her to feel it fully and connect her breath while feeling it. When she stayed with the feeling, rather than trying to "make" it go away, it dissipated on its own. Using these new words allowed her to have a different relationship to the feelings she was having and it was easier to breathe with them.

After that, her stories calmed down. They became quieter and easier to deal with. And pretty soon she was able to see that all the hot and jumpy stuff was really only energy. Instead of reviewing and reliving all the old stories in her head, the entire ten-part Netflix series of the times she felt she was a fraud and not enough, she realized she could instead use her energy to be creative and find a solution to the challenge at hand.

In the last chapter, we talked about intentions and how making simple declarations about how you want to feel can change your brain chemistry and change your energy. Together, the woman and I worked on some new intentions she could try at work. The next time she felt her face growing hot during a meeting, she began taking deeper and smoother breaths. And she repeated to herself: *I'm worthy and capable.*

Even if this seems overly simplistic to you, this technique works time and time again.

The meeting went on.

She did not feel hot and jumpy.

Her face did not turn red.

In subsequent breathwork sessions, we continued to practice conscious breathing and intention setting, and very soon, when the woman was in an office meeting and felt the hot and jumpy sensation inside her, she found the strength to shift her energy enough to speak up—and shift the conversation too. She was proactive. "I hear you," she said, and, "I think if we tried this."

Eventually, as we did more breathwork and she began practicing at home, the woman came up with ways to reimagine her concept of what an office meeting was. Rather than seeing this aspect of her professional life as pure torture, she began to think of her office meetings as simply brainstorming sessions. They were a chance to toss out ideas and solve problems that needed solving. And, even better, she began to see that she was *good* at brainstorming.

Rather than letting her energy go toward flushes and self-judgment stories, she used her energy to be creative. She figured out that her "panic flushes" were actually energy rushes.

What if we could all shift our experiences that way? Rather than telling ourselves, "Oh no, oh no, oh no, *here comes PANIC!*" we could instead think, "Hey, look, *I can really feel the energy flowing now.*"

Drama is Optional

Often, when we have physical reactions—our faces turn red, our skin sweats, or we get sick to our stomachs—we feel like there is something "wrong" with us. As a young mom, I often hit code-red and was overwhelmed by my own big feelings as well as everybody else's. Part of what led me to feeling anxious and tight was never knowing what was coming next. My feelings were unpredictable, so I bounced around as I reacted to them.

A rush of energy can come without notice. You can be feeling peaceful and quiet one minute and suddenly, your emotions flip when you hear something upsetting or drop a box on your foot and feel tremendous pain. Your energy shifts immediately and becomes fast and jarring. You react with a code-red stress response that escalates your adrenaline and cortisol levels.

Whether it's physical pain or emotional pain, energy rushes can unhinge us. This is why so many people are afraid of their feelings, the way I used to be afraid of mine. What causes us to be afraid of feelings is that we don't feel like we can control them.

They come when we aren't ready for them.

What breathwork teaches us is that feelings are energy and energy is natural. Human beings are really like radio towers. What comes through us constantly changes. The signals and channels continue to change, along with the music. As soon as you understand this, you will become more comfortable with the sensations that come with emotion rushing into your body. And once you learn not to attach drama to those sensations, you can achieve more mastery over your energy—and feelings.

Drama is optional.

Energy just shows up.

Sometimes energy feels heavy, wiry, light, flowy, jumpy, or tight. But, it is just passing through and will move on. There's no reason to judge that energy or give it labels, good or bad. And there is no point in creating soap operas in your head that connect these sensations to other times in your life when you felt out of control or afraid or anxious.

Instead of panic or drama, you learn in breathwork to experience a feeling coming on and say, "Oh, isn't that interesting, there's that energy sensation again." You learn to continue breathing with the energy as it comes, the same way the pregnant woman I wrote about in the last chapter learned to be okay with her fear and allowed it to come and go. Each breath could release fear, rather than keeping it around like a possession you can't possibly part with.

The same thing is true for people who suffer from chronic pain, the subject of my next chapter. Pain and fear can go hand in hand. Rather than going into code-red every time you have an uncomfortable sensation, and reacting by holding your breath and triggering the fight-or-flight response in your body, you can stay calm and balanced by flowing with your breath.

Breathwork teaches a whole new approach to feelings. By fully experiencing your emotions and the sensations that come with them, and not reacting, you are able to be with your feelings, manage them, and choose how to respond to them.

Why?

You've gotten out of your head, and out of storytelling mode. You know whatever comes up in breathwork, you are ready to process.

In other words, you are present.

Suddenly your experience of being alive—of literally *being you*—is free and clear of additives. Free of drama. Free of junk. Free of all the stuff and stories you've made up and repeated to yourself over your lifetime.

It's just you and your breath, and you are riding a wave of energy.

Now let's see how big and dramatic you can be. Take a moment to produce your best and biggest sigh. Beautiful. Let's try another. This time, see if you can let all of your frustrations out in your next big dramatic sigh. Louder! Good! We all have lots of ways to release energy—and lots of different sighs inside us. See how many you've got. Play around, have fun with your sighs.

Try a silent sigh with no drama.

Try a dramatic long, low, deep sigh.

Try giggling while you sigh. (It's possible, it really is!)

Keep breathing, inhale through your nose and exhale from your mouth. With every exhale, try a different sigh and see how each one feels. Notice how you feel inside after your tenth breath.

Start your own repertoire of sighs. You'll need them!

The Big Kahuna

Eventually, you will relax more around these surges. You might say things like, "Oh, that's energy coming through me right now. I'm going to get present by breathing into my belly." Breath is the superhighway to present moment awareness. In the present moment, you can be relaxed and creative, rather than reactive and tense.

When you learn to connect your breath, lots of practical things can happen—your professional life becomes easier, your relationships improve, the world seems better— because your spiritual being is finally being spoken with, listened to, cared for, and understood. Your posture improves. You handle things differently.

Breath brings wisdom and strength.

You begin to feel more confident and balanced. You begin to *feel* more, period, because you aren't afraid of your energy anymore. You know whatever comes up, however strong the wave, whatever happens, you can cope. Every time you fall off-center, you have a place to go—your breath. And the energy is you!

Breath
brings
wisdom
and
strength.

CHAPTER 4

LETTING GO AND BECOMING FLOW

A sudden, sharp pain can be so jolting. I remember one experience so vividly. My kids were still little and I was running late and racing around the grocery store, trying to get some food for dinner. I was wearing flip-flops and totally in my head—not paying attention. A big wooden crate of fruit was just sitting there, quietly, and my toes plowed right into it. Really hard. I mean, *so so so hard*. The pain was immediate and excruciating.

I froze.

I heard a voice in my head.

Practice what you preach!

I had been doing breathwork for four or five years by then. So, I had the ropes down. I started breathing in the middle of the grocery store and allowed an incredible big wave of emotion and pain to crash over me, and kept breathing with it.

Within a few breaths, the pain was gone.

I looked up, kind of amazed. The fear and upset were over. Usually the pain when I stubbed my toe would last for a day or two, and it would just kind of travel with me. But rather than limping in a wounded way down all the aisles of the store, I felt okay. I didn't even wake up the next day with a throbbing foot. I didn't even get a bruise.

All Kinds of Pain

There are different kinds of pain. Sometimes it's mental or spiritual. Sometimes it's physical, like when your body has an injury. Usually, in addition to the physical pain sensation you feel, there is an emotional response. It accompanies the shock and upset over your injury. Like me and my stubbed toe, or the woman I found injured on the ski slopes after a wipe-out, physical pain triggers a feeling of helplessness, a sense of being out of control and sometimes an overwrought fear. "This will kill me!"

Only part of my distress in the grocery store was actually happening in my foot. The other parts were all the thoughts racing around my head.

"Oh no, what happened?"

"Did I break my toe?"

"Will I be in pain all week?"

"I'm such a clod. It's all my fault."

This boils down to two kinds of pain: physical pain and story/emotional pain. Our central nervous system does not know the difference between them. They have the same vibration. When we are injured, we often go into shallow-breathing mode, taking shorter breaths or holding our breath, whether the pain is physical or mental.

Eventually, after we calm down and breathe consciously, the physical pain is more bearable. The more we can relax and breathe, the more manageable physical pain becomes, particularly if we don't wrap a story around it.

Mind Over Pain

I learned more than I ever wanted to know about spines and something called "stenosis" when I was going from doctor to doctor, trying to find relief for my neck pain.

One thing I finally came to accept is that most people over the age of thirty or thirty-five have something called "stenosis." Their range of motion is limited by tightness. An MRI or X-ray will usually give a doctor an explanation for pain. The bigger mystery is that most people with spinal stenosis and arthritis go through life without pain.

Yes.

They are pain free.

That was the discovery of a physician of physical rehabilitation at NYU, Dr. John Sarno. People can function with crushed disks and twisted spines. Most people with serious spinal conditions do.

His conclusion: Stenosis doesn't cause pain.

Dr. Sarno's book, *Mind Over Back Pain*, changed the conversation about back pain and back surgery—and changed life for many chronic sufferers. If you've had back pain, you know how miserable and debilitating it can be. Dr. Sarno was the first respected Western medical expert to reach a mainstream audience with this piece of ancient wisdom: the mind and body are connected.

Bottom line?

The brain generates the pain signal, not the body.

Therefore, the mind is the source of the pain.

My own journey through chronic pain had made this crystal clear to me. When clients come to my practice because they have physical pains that traditional Western medical treatments haven't helped, I tell them about my neck. I've been there. I know.

The pain feels so real.

It's so urgent—and *loud*.

Sometimes it's hard to think or move.

And you've tried everything under the sun.

So, how can it be "all in my head"?

Think about that phrase for a second. *All in your head.* It was probably coined by a skeptic trying to be funny. Except, wait, it couldn't be more true! Originally, my neck pain may have started with a physical strain or injury. My brain sent a pain signal to my neck. This is what the mind is supposed to do, to let the body know it needs to be careful and not re-injure that hurt place.

Sometimes, though, the signal stays on *even after the injury is long gone*. The mind just hasn't gotten the news that you're better. Or the mind wants to get your attention about some other "pain." This is what creates habitual pain or chronic pain. When it is presenting itself in the back or neck, people become truly afraid to move at all. They are afraid of having even *more* pain or causing further damage.

And we know what being afraid does to us.

We get tighter.

We get constricted.

We don't think clearly.

We begin living in fear.

It's a vicious cycle.

Western medical doctors might prescribe a tranquilizer or pain medication at this point. This sort of medication numbs you. It's just a bandage. And after a while, the medication wears off or stops working. And you find yourself, as I did, needing to double your dose. Or you might find yourself truly addicted to the medication, which just compounds all the things you now have to deal with.

Drugs might not be the answer.

So, where do you turn?

The mind is the place to start working on chronic pain. That's where the signal is being sent—from your head, your heart, your buried feelings. In my breathwork practice, I have seen amazing things happen as soon as a client even opens to the idea that they can "feel" their pain fully, all the sensations, and "release" themselves from the pain cycle. The pain signal is broken up. Breathing through pain is a way to tell your mind, "Hey, thank you for keeping me safe and you don't need to do that anymore!"

Getting the hang of this can require coaching.

That's where breathworkers like me come in.

All in My Head?

I've seen clients have immediate results from just one breathwork session. But if you have been experiencing long-term chronic pain, your muscles and connective tissue can change shape from being held in a pattern of tension for so long. Some tissues can lengthen, others shorten. As a breathworker, it's my honor to help clients open up their breath pattern and begin breathing into the tight areas to break the pattern of how the body is holding pain.

In the case of my neck pain, relief wasn't immediate. I had lots of stuff to release, lots of stories I'd told myself about needing to be perfect, about how I wasn't enough. Those feelings and energy had been stuffed down inside me for years, hidden away.

The pain in my neck wanted to be heard, and understood. My neck pain was a signal. A loud and blaring signal. It was trying to tell me something.

What was it saying?

Pay attention!

Are you listening, Lauren?

There is
power in
vulnerability.

For me, it took a combination of physical therapy, yoga, meditation, and breathwork to finally listen to what my mind and body wanted me to hear—like, how I was shoving my voice and my needs down. It was unspoken emotion. Once I started to breathe into those feelings and speak my needs, my neck began to open up! I released the tension and stuck energy.

Like many of my clients, I started breathwork for relief from physical pain and wound up with a lot more, making a leap to a whole new way of living. I shifted from a tight shallow chest breath to a full diaphragmatic breath. I began to see that I had lived my life in fear of not being enough and not being worthy.

And I made the shift from fear to love.

My body still likes to tell me things—and I've learned to listen. When I experience tightness, when my neck or my knee or shoulder is hurting, I go to my breath first and ask that area what it needs. When I breathe, it helps bring wisdom in. That is one thing I trust now, most of all: The body has tremendous wisdom. Let yours speak to you.

Here's an exercise to try. If you had trouble getting your belly to rise while inhaling during the exercise in Chapter Two, this could help you. For the rest of you, this is a way to become more open and flowing.

First, listen to your body and find its tight spots. Your body might be telling you that your belly is tight. You could start by using your fingertips to massage around your belly to find some tight spots while connecting your breath. As you breathe and massage, you'll start to feel the tight spots getting looser.

Now see if you can find other places to open. Work your fingers up to your chest muscles—and onto your shoulders, neck, face, and scalp. The looser and more relaxed your body is, the more open your breath will be.

Stuck in Neutral

There are other forms of chronic pain.

"I can't get out of bed."

"I can't get out of my bathtub."

"I'm stuck."

Depression can feel like heavy, thick, and sluggish energy. It can leave people feeling tired, flat, burdened, weighed down.

Sometimes, you're barely able to move, work, or get out of the house. When a client comes to me because they are suffering from "chronic" depression, the first thing I do is stop using the "d-word." It's powerful and loaded. And it can even trigger a person back into an episode just by thinking about it.

How does energy become stuck?

We just don't want to feel our feelings. We just don't. We suppress and tamp them down. For many people, there's a lot of fear in feeling. Your mind says, "No way! I'm not feeling that!" Your mind sits in judgment of the feeling, decides it's bad. You might feel sad, but your inner critic says it's wrong to feel sorry for yourself, or crying is for babies. You might feel angry, but you have self-judgment about that and think it's wrong to feel angry. So, you don't allow yourself to have that feeling.

When we were little, not many of us were encouraged to express our feelings—to shout or cry or get angry. Even after we've grown up, the voices of our parents continue in our heads. The minute we feel sad or want to cry, we say to ourselves, "Stop that crying!"

Or we offer bribes: "If you stop that crying, I'll give you a piece of cake, a glass of wine, a new toy." We reward ourselves for tamping those "wrong" feelings down. That's how overeating starts. That's how addictions can start, and where retail therapy begins sucking the cash from your bank account. You have a feeling you don't want to feel. When you suppress it, you reward yourself with unlimited junk food. Or you reward yourself with a drug or alcohol binge, which temporarily numbs the feeling you think is bad.

Breathwork for depression or any kind of stuck energy is really helpful because you're moving what has been stuck. When I work with someone who is depressed, I get them to deepen their inhale gradually, just a little fraction. When they do that, even a tiny bit, it can make a difference, because they've opened a little of their constriction.

Even just a little movement, a little opening, can be the key.

Then I really get them moving; when they are lying on the floor on a futon and their breath is flowing, I get them kicking and pounding. I've seen depressed people kick and pound so hard that I thought, "Oh my goodness, they're either going to break their fists or the futon!"

And then, suddenly, they are giggling or laughing. Once their breath begins flowing and their body is moving, the sensation of that flowing and moving energy is very powerful. That's why exercise, like fast walking, running, or swimming, is so effective for depression. Your body moves, your breath moves, and your energy moves with it.

I have an exercise for you now. It's fun—trust me—because it allows you to have a big, beautiful tantrum that gets your energy flowing. First, you create an intention. If you are feeling stuck or depressed, an intention that could work might be: *I am energetic and flowing*, or *I am happy*. As you're breathing, allow this intention to be repeated in your mind.

If you are sitting in a chair, start stomping your feet on the floor and punch your fists up into the air over your head, as if you are punching the sky. Like you're having an adult tantrum! If you are lying on the sofa or a yoga mat, you can run in place with your feet on the floor and pound your fists on two pillows on the mat. While doing this, turn your head side-to-side like you're saying "no, no, no" and make a sound or tone; vocal toning is using your voice to create vibrations in the body.

Tone *AHHHH* with everything you've got. That's right. Keep going. Be as loud as you can! Toning the vowels of the alphabet, A-E-I-O-U, helps clear our energetic pathways. *AHHHH*, in particular, helps clear the heart.

Go on, try it.

Wake the neighbors!

Repeating your intention while moving stuck energy allows you to do a couple of important things. First, it reconnects you to the place where you are already happy. Second, it helps you begin to remember what it is like to be energetic, flowing, and happy, creating a feeling you can return to, again and again, whenever you are feeling stuck.

One of my clients who was struggling with depression used to say, "Lauren, you're always in my head! I hear you guiding me!" In the morning, if she woke up and couldn't get out of bed, she remembered I had taught her to start with just a tiny breath, an inhalation, then make it bigger, and bigger, and bigger. Then she'd start moving— kicking, pounding, maybe a little toning, *AHHHH*. After twenty or thirty connected breaths while repeating her intention in her head—*I am energetic, I am flowing, I am happy*—this exercise never failed her. She would always get herself to work that day.

Let Go and Let Flow

Control does not bring happiness, or freedom, or a sense of aliveness. Control brings tightness and constriction. It is a fearful response to life. It is only by learning how to stop controlling, and by relaxing, that you are able to be in the flow—the flow of life, the flow of change.

The French philosopher and Buddhist monk, Matthieu Ricard, has a great way of explaining this idea. He says when we try to control life and live in a self-contained and controlled way, it is like we are trying to build a stunning boat that will carry us across a river. We work really hard on that boat—we make it beautiful, give it new gadgets and teak decks. We polish the hull and the shiny brass. We pour all our attention and energy into that boat. We make sure it looks perfect, like the way we fixate on our own appearances or our families.

Ricard offers another way to live:

Don't worry about the boat. Let it go. Let go of perfection.

Be the river beneath it.

And when you are breathing and flowing, that's where you are. You let go of the boat and join the river. You become the flow. You open to a state of being that is always there for you—wherever you are, whatever you are facing. Letting go means joining the river of light, the life force, a rushing stream of energy and unconditional love. This powerful energy runs through us and *is* us. Even someone who has spent years in chronic pain can let go and flow.

It can happen in a second.

It can happen without thinking about it.

You just breathe.

Sometimes people start laughing. Or smiling. Or crying. Flow can be the flow of tears. No big deal. *Let those tears come gushing. We all have tears! So, let's really have them!*

We are healthiest when we are open and flowing. We are more flexible, more able to dance, more in the moment and present. Our energy feels yummy. When we try to control our emotions all the time, when we are holding on and trying not to cry, it will leak out in other ways. If the energy has trouble flowing, it becomes uncomfortable. The tightness of holding in our feelings can become painful.

Learning to feel those feelings—fully—and being okay with everything that arises with them takes practice. Connecting with our inner wisdom and all our feelings, and learning to be with them and to breathe with them, is key to becoming the flow.

Releasing and letting go allows us to become fully present. We become aware. We become our authentic selves. This is how you begin tossing out the stories, the labels, and everything else that isn't what is true inside you.

This is emotional mastery.

Control does not bring happiness.

Being Present

When you are telling yourself a story—"I'm not good enough"—you are not present. When you are reacting to fear of feeling your emotions, you are not present either.

Why do we need to overthink things and make everything more complicated? We don't. It's really simple. There are things you can do, right now, to become more present.

Here's a way to start:

Feel the temperature of the room on your skin.

Feel the cool air entering your nose and the warm air leaving your nose.

Smell the air where you're sitting.

Taste the taste in your mouth and then gently swallow.

Listen for the farthest sound you can hear.

Feel your shoulders relaxing on every exhale.

Breathe into where your sit-bones touch the seat cushion.

Every conscious breath brings you back to the present moment.

Answers come more easily when your brain isn't churning.

Answers come, like a gift.

Every breath gives you a do-over.

When you're present with yourself, you feel connected. There is no fear, only a sense of responding to life as it unfolds. When you're present with yourself, you also begin to see how easy things could be. How free you can feel. How unburdened. You want to start letting go more and more, and releasing the baggage you've been carrying around forever. It's not hard to do!

You just have to say *YES* to the breath and let go of the stories.

Baggage Drop

We carry so much emotional baggage around with us. We often don't even know all the stuff we are carrying. Baggage in the form of expectations, things our parents or society told us we needed. Ways of life and conventions we've inherited.

With breathwork, you learn to free yourself of expectations. You begin to let go, and become lighter and freer. You feel more and more like yourself and have the courage to follow your heart more.

In my early breathwork sessions, I let go of perfection. I learned it was okay to be a beautiful mess. I didn't need perfect hair and a perfect blow-out—even though those things are still fun! I didn't need to be in control of every possible scenario. I learned it was okay to cry, to giggle, to laugh really loud. I even learned to roar. Before I started breathwork, I was a pressure cooker and the lid was on *tight*. No crying allowed. *AND NO ROARING!*

You know, there's strength in being a beautiful mess, because it's liberating for everybody around you. It allows them to be beautiful messes too.

And it spreads the message: there's power in vulnerability.

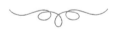

There is
strength
in being a
beautiful
mess.

CHAPTER 5

THE AUTHENTIC YOU

We are creatures of habit. We get into patterns that make us feel comfortable and safe. Habits reassure us and, sometimes, come to define us. They can also be numbing, many times keeping us from living as our authentic selves.

I didn't fully understand how routines affected us until I went through breathwork training. I attended a retreat where everyone in my class was asked to fast for twenty-four hours. In our everyday life, food can become a habit too. When you eat the same things in the same way, it's like your tongue goes to sleep and can't wake up. You stop really tasting anything. After twenty-four hours of not eating, our breathwork teacher gave us each a fresh strawberry to smell.

Wow. What a sweet, fruity smell! My toes were curling. You should try it sometime. When you smell a strawberry after you haven't eaten for twenty-four hours, it's an amazing experience. *It smells like a celebration.*

When
the child
deep inside
us heals,
our spirit
blossoms.

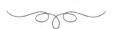

After we smelled and swooned over our strawberries, we were invited to eat them.

What was that like?

An explosion in my mouth. Goodness, sweetness, muskiness, and juiciness. I thought I might pass out from pleasure. The taste was so vibrant and powerful. And that feeling has stayed with me. I never want to eat a strawberry again in the same old way.

I want to really taste it.

I want to fully experience it.

I want that strawberry to explode in my mouth!

Even today when I see a strawberry on my plate, I remember that life-changing experience and I try to recreate it. I try to taste the strawberry without that thick fog of habit and routine. It's the way I want to feel about everything I do—living authentically and relishing every moment.

How can we all do that?

By waking up and embracing the joys of life, negotiating everyday stresses and pressures, and letting go of stories and memories that keep us distracted. The way to be fully awake to a strawberry, or anything else on your plate, is to be *present*.

Breathwork is a highway to being fully awake and present. It is a way to hit the refresh button by scraping away the extraneous thoughts in your mind. As children, we experience an authentic self until it becomes buried in layers of adult expectations, memories, wounds, and obligations. We get lost in our own ideas about who we are "supposed" to be. When you start breathwork and begin shedding baggage and reconnecting to your authentic self, it feels a little like eating after a long fast. You wake up. You are buzzing with energy. You don't feel you need anything more.

Your heart is full.

Your body is relaxed.

You are fully oxygenated and fully present, smelling the air and feeling the moment. After their first session, people often say things like, "I feel so connected" or "Wow, this is the best I've felt in a long time." And they say they want to feel that way more often.

When the child deep inside us heals, our spirit blossoms. I've seen a sixty-eight-year-old woman buy a skateboard and start riding it. I've had clients who decide to quit a soul-killing job or move to the beach. One man decided to learn how to fly a plane.

This chapter is about what happens when you start letting go. You reconnect to your authentic self. When you do that, no matter how long it's been, the change can be profound. If you are in a long-term relationship, things get refreshed. Your connection feels alive again. There's more to talk about.

Suddenly there's more time for adventure and play.

Best of all, there's way more love.

"I'm a Whole Being!"

One of my first clients was a man in his seventies, a distinguished psychiatrist with an assortment of degrees, published research, prizes, and acclaim. He also had a serious heart condition and some pulmonary issues.

When he arrived at my home office, he was huffing and puffing from having climbed a steep set of stairs to get to my front door. Once I'd greeted him, there were more stairs for him to climb. In those days, we lived in an old 1917 house and my breathwork space was on the third floor. Watching my new client going up the stairs, I worried he might not make it. And he barely did. He had to keep stopping to catch his breath. Those flights of stairs were like climbing Kilimanjaro with a polished oak railing.

Once we sat down together and he recovered, he told me about his heart condition and began listing all the medications he was taking. He had a big personality and told me about his work and career, the important medical boards he sat on, the prizes he had won. I could tell these things were a significant part of his identity. At the same time, he looked sallow and worn out as he listed them.

We worked together every two weeks. Arriving for his session, he'd take his time as he climbed the stairs and then would throw himself into breathwork. After he learned the basics of breathwork and connecting his breath, the real magic began: he connected with himself. He began releasing energy and experiencing things that had been buried inside him for a long time. Sure, he had been in some sort of psychotherapy or psychoanalysis himself, as most professionals in the field of mental health have. He was familiar with his childhood wounds and early impressions of the world that had informed his adult life. These were facts he could recite, but not emotions. Once he got connected to himself, he realized that old feelings from his boyhood were still inside him.

His father had actively disliked him. His mother never had time for him. As a boy, he hadn't been given the love he needed. He'd been neglected and ignored. This left him feeling deprived and sad. And that stayed with him. He was a man who had carried his boyhood loneliness around his whole life. Each week, he arrived at my door with a smile, but there was also a cloud of sorrow around him.

We all have an authentic self—a core, a spirit, a soul. No matter how long we've been away from it, or forgotten it was there, that authentic self is still with us like a faithful friend. It is always waiting for us. And once we reconnect to it, we feel more grounded and safe and whole.

My client connected to that place inside himself and began breathing into the layers of emotional wounds, the childhood sadness and loneliness, and began releasing it. The color began to appear in his face. By the end of the second month, I noticed he had less trouble going up the stairs. He didn't need to stop to catch his breath.

By the third month, he began releasing huge chunks of stuck energy. Things kept coming up. He realized how much music meant to him, and how creative he was—something that had been buried inside him. When his sense of loneliness came up, he kept breathing and gave himself the love his parents never had.

And this love began healing him.

"I'm not a heart patient, I'm a whole being!" he called out one day.

His complexion wasn't sallow anymore, even before a breathwork session. He told me that his circulation was improving. His cardiologist had reduced his heart medications.

By the fourth month of breathwork, he was playing guitar with friends. In one breath session, in the middle of releasing energy, he suddenly began singing "Ring of Fire"—the Johnny Cash song—at the top of his lungs. He cried hard and the tears washed the years of emotional gunk away.

He became clear and vibrant after that. He was radiant, alive, and glittering—and roaring with life! I marveled too, and felt so grateful for his work and for him. What an honor it was to sit back and watch this man come alive. By then, when he came to his session, he practically bounded up the stairs.

Sometimes people come to me because they think they are dying, or have been told by a doctor they are. When they connect with their breath, they see they've been afraid of living. And they see how a medical diagnosis could be just a story that creates more fear, more tightness, anxiety, and stress. A diagnosis is just a bunch of words that people put meaning to. Once they experience their authentic self—and are free of stories—they start seeing that anything is possible.

As soon as you get a whiff of your aliveness, and your wholeness, you don't want to go back. Your courage grows and your desire to keep showing up as your authentic self becomes very strong.

We all have an authentic self—a core, a spirit, a soul.

Breathwork and Relationships

A number of my clients have come to see me when traditional couples therapy didn't do the trick. They felt stuck in an unhappy place. Or they just weren't moving as fast as they wanted to a better place. Sometimes their psychotherapist sent them to me, or a friend recommended me.

These couples sit across from me tight and constricted and sometimes fuming and angry. One of them will explain, "She's driving me crazy and I feel like I'm never enough!" Or they sit in silence with heavy energy in the room. Their emotions have been tamped down, left to suffocate or smolder.

We talk for a bit and I have them create intentions and they begin to breathe. Even if they are shallow breathers and constricted, one session can open them up enough to begin to change things. Nine times out of ten, by the end of their first session, the couple is holding hands while they're breathing. They have gotten closer to their authentic selves. They have begun to remember why they are together and what they mean to each other. They've gotten past the words, the fear, and they've gotten back to love.

Eventually, in time, they open up more and more. A lot of people are in relationships where their egos are running the show. It's hard for them to be vulnerable. But in time, they can say things out loud, things that have been buried inside them and, afterward, they breathe together in a session. I can't overstate how healing this can be, and how helpful it is for a couple that is struggling to find their connection again. Really, it's all about moving from fear to love again.

Most of the time, people haven't fallen out of love. They are just clinging to fear. Like everybody else, their childhood experiences between the ages of zero and seven affect their marriage and the way they connect with other people. The kind of relationship their parents had—and the kind of household they were raised in—sets the stage for what they will later think of as "normal." This idea of normal will define the way we act in a relationship. It sets our expectations.

If you grew up in a family where people were always yelling at each other, that behavior will seem normal to you. You may think that's just how things are supposed to be. Your picture of "love" includes screaming at each other. And when you start talking about this with your partner, sharing your childhood feelings and fears, how hard it was to live in a house of yelling, you might discover you've been yelling the way your parents did. "Oh my God, I'm doing the same thing!"

In breathwork, you can learn to catch yourself before the yelling starts. You start to notice the habitual patterns.

You learn to regroup, take a breath, take a walk, whatever you need to do in order to find your wisdom and then respond to your partner in a different way. On this very practical level, breathwork can shift behavior. It gives you a way to be more comfortable with being vulnerable, rather than raging and yelling, and you're able to show up in a relationship in a higher and healthier way. Breath creates space for you to respond from your highest self.

Vulnerability is Strength

We're all vulnerable. To be aware and alive is to understand our profound vulnerability. We're living on a planet that is hurtling through space and, on top of that, if you're in a committed relationship, you are traveling through life hitched to another human being!

What is more vulnerable than a relationship? Because while we are hurtling through space, we are also continuing to grow and change. Each day, hour, or year of a relationship can be different. Sometimes you're hot and heavy for each other and sometimes you're cold and dry. This is just how relationships roll.

All relationships ebb and flow like the ocean. But change can bring uncertainty and fear. *Has he stopped loving me? Are we still a happy couple? Is she bored?*

If you're not comfortable with being vulnerable, you might try to keep things going exactly as they are, as long as possible, even if that means connecting to a story or connecting to fear, rather than creating a deeper and stronger connection that is authentic. If a couple can experience their vulnerability together, they find their power and true strength in the moment.

They will be soft and strong at the same time.

Because this paradox is true: Vulnerability is strength. We are strongest when we're vulnerable. People who act like they're never vulnerable—and never admit weakness— are the most brittle of all. Even their breath is tight. They are pretending to themselves, acting, faking it, and have sealed up their authentic selves. Because we really don't know much, do we? Some of the strongest and wisest people I know are completely comfortable saying, "I really don't know." I love it when anybody says that.

And I try to stay vulnerable myself. I try to wake up every day in "beginner mind" as they say in Zen. Yes, here I am, giving you all this advice and being my expert-self as a breathwork trainer and teacher, and at the same time, I know how much I still have to learn. It's crucial to live that way. Each day, as soon as I open my eyes, stretch my body, and breathe, I am opening myself up for a new day, new experiences, and new ways of being. I am ready to learn something new.

When you get to that place of openness, when you are soft and strong, you can ride the waves of emotion and all the transitions and changes that come with being alive. And come with all relationships. You learn to be okay with shifts in energy and feeling.

And why is that important?

If you are able to be vulnerable, you allow the people around you to be vulnerable—and allow them to change and grow. With that, your relationship becomes a living and breathing and growing thing. That's when the a-ha moments begin. Clarity comes. Insights come. You begin to create a new way to be together.

Does that guarantee you will "work things out" and stay together? No. It does not guarantee that. But, if one of you decides to leave, it could be *with love*, not drama. It guarantees if you do grow apart, you could help yourself and your partner take a step forward, and embrace something new that neither one of you thought you could.

Growth brings uncertainty.

Growth brings more vulnerability.

Growth also brings excitement, aliveness, honesty, and profound connection.

Intimacy and Breath

Couples often come to see me because one or both of them is having trouble being intimate. Some people just don't really enjoy sex. I hear it in my practice. They want to enjoy it, or maybe they once did, and they sense they are now missing out on something great and don't know how to get the feeling back.

Usually that lack of enjoyment comes down to an insecurity or a fear. They are scared of how they look naked or worry about how they'll be perceived. They don't like their breasts or bellies. They worry that they aren't pleasing their partners or they won't be able to perform well. They also have memories that come up—stories—that get in the way of fully experiencing and enjoying a sexual encounter.

Sometimes they aren't even aware of their fear or anxiety. Instead, they talk about all the special conditions they need in order to feel sexually aroused. They need the lights shut off. Or they need a lot of warmth and heat; they can't have sex if the room is cold. They want more control, which is a tip-off that they feel scared and vulnerable. There is sometimes so much tightness and constriction around sex—and often everything else in their life—they've stopped really breathing as soon as their partner strokes their arm or has that look in their eye.

That look scares them. They might feel hunted or preyed upon. They feel vulnerable and fearful. *That look* means they'll need to take off their clothes. It means being physically and emotionally vulnerable.

To understand how much breathing can change things for them, I'll tell you how people in my practice have said that when they're consciously breathing, one gentle caress on their arm can send them into an orgasm.

Pleasure is healing.

So is being alive in the moment, and being present with your partner.

How can you get there? Breath is a path to every aspect of being fully alive. It teaches us how to relax and feel pleasure when we are not in control. Even the word "respiration" tells us that. Respiration, in Latin, can mean breathing in spirit, to come alive again! If every breath makes us feel alive, just imagine what breath could be like when you're having sex.

Here's something to warm you up: Take in a full breath and let it out with a slow, low *MMMMM* tone. Now another breath, full and deep, and let it out with another slow *MMMMM*. One more time. Take a breath and this time, let it out with *YUMMMM*.

Breath and sound together are magic.

Pleasure is healing.

Ecstasy is Necessary

Over the years, I've worked with lots of therapists and have given breathwork sessions at psychotherapy conferences.

Traditional therapy and breathwork can work well in collaboration. Sometimes you can only get so far with "talk therapy." You could get stuck in one place. Sometimes a therapist could become stuck with a patient and think that breathwork could unstick them.

Therapists have said to me that one private breathwork session, or even a group breath session, is like ten therapy sessions. It's a shortcut, like when you are playing the game of Chutes & Ladders and you get to skip ahead. Breathing has a way of wordlessly accessing the subconscious stuff, which is kept under lock and key. When you're connecting your breath in a relaxed body, you feel safe to allow your memories and emotions to come up.

When they do, the rest can be easier than you'd ever guess. Experience those feelings and memories fully and completely. Just breathe with them and process and integrate them until they become energy and you are back in the flow.

Flow is juicy!

Once you are shedding the stories and fear, and beginning to live in a connected way with your authentic self, things will change and flow. You start listening to your instincts, your senses, and your heart—like the psychiatrist who belted out "Ring of Fire" in my breathwork space. "Ring of Fire" was his call to life. It was the song of his aliveness and renewed spirit.

Being authentic means being you, not just following the rules and conventions of society or your peer group to the point of numbness. It means listening to yourself and knowing yourself, and who you really are. For example, rather than telling your body when to eat, because that has been decided by your family, you can do things differently.

After years of eating three meals a day and believing rigid routine was important, now I eat only when I'm hungry.

My body has led me to that decision. This didn't happen overnight. And it wasn't something I forced on myself. It happened when I started listening to my body. While I ate Ho Hos and Twinkies as a kid, I couldn't imagine having them now. But I'm definitely down for a decadent piece of dark chocolate.

Who are you deep down?

Where does that authentic you want to play?

Take five minutes to breathe in a quiet place, seamlessly connecting your inhale to your exhale. Have a pen and paper or your journal nearby, because I have some questions for you—and for you only. The only person reading your answers is you. Try to release that inner critic. Try not to edit yourself. Be completely free.

I want you to think about a perfect day. And by that, I mean *your* perfect day. Where are you waking up? What does the room look like and feel like? Are you alone or with someone? What are you having for breakfast? What will you do on this perfect day; how will you fill the minutes and hours?

Sit on the beach?

Take a bike ride or a hike?

How does the day look, feel, and smell?

How would the day end?

Go for it, really have fun with this, and be as detailed as you like. How often do you get a chance to really think about something like this? The next step is even more interesting, in a way. What does your perfect day tell you about yourself—and what you need more of in life? How do you begin to create this for yourself?

The road to knowing ourselves begins with openness. I have learned from my clients and from my own experience with breathwork that we are all curious about who we really are when the "shoulds" and "coulds" are gone. We have lots of masks, different personas for different settings and occasions.

If you peeled off all those masks, what's underneath? Who is there? What song would you sing? And once you've sung your song—or sung a bunch of songs—you can make some other discoveries.

Answering these questions could require you to be courageous. Listening carefully to the answers might require some courage too. Set aside fears about what you may discover.

There is only one authentic you.

CHAPTER 6

LOVING YOURSELF

My grandmother always accepted me exactly as I was. When I was little and always racing around and having meltdowns, she never scolded me for being emotional or said things like, "Big girls don't cry!" Instead, she fed my imagination with wonderful stories about princesses and magical kingdoms. As I got older and entered my awkward teen years, she never tried to fix my hair or make me wear clothes I didn't like.

When I reached adulthood, she called every weekend to hear how I was and celebrated my professional successes. She was thrilled about my marriage. Her love was *unconditional*.

What does that mean?

She just loved me.

She loved me as I was.

I didn't really understand how different unconditional love felt from other kinds of love until my wonderful grandmother died. Unconditional love seemed to die with her.

I cried so hard when I lost her. I felt so alone. I didn't just miss my sweet and sassy grandmother. I missed the way she made me feel—accepted, worthy, 100 percent okay in every way. I cried because I thought nobody would ever love me like that again.

Her love was soft and flowing and constantly there. She had known me forever, since I was a little girl who had meltdowns and also danced and played dress up. My husband and friends loved me, but they only knew the woman I became, the one who kept the trains running and who didn't always speak her mind or live from her heart.

They knew that *woman*, but not the playful little girl deep inside.

When I started breathwork, I cried again thinking of my grandmother and what she had given me. She was so warm and fun and amazing. Her love was so strong and unwavering. And then, one day, I discovered there was somebody on earth who could give me that same kind of unconditional love.

Me.

What I discovered was that the most healing and sustaining love doesn't come from outside. You don't have to wait around for it, like an external prize or reward. Breathwork taught me that unconditional love was available to me all the time, wherever I went, whatever I did.

It was inside me all along.

What I felt inside, unconditional love for myself, was flowing and warm and soft and constantly there, just the way my grandmother's love had been. Breathwork did that for me. And that's huge! So, this chapter is about how you can learn to have total acceptance and respect for yourself. A place where you feel safe and loved.

Understanding Love

All sorts of things shift as soon as you begin shifting your breath. For starters, it brings a much keener awareness of your own energy. When you connect your breath, you begin to learn how energy feels and how it flows. You begin to understand the words "open and flowing"—and what they literally mean and feel like. Very quickly, you are able to spot your tightness.

Until they begin breathing, most of my clients don't realize they've been in fear-mode or semi-fear-mode a great part of their lives.

We all know about fear. I think we're kind of trained by society and by our families to understand it—intimately. We're warned about dangers and diseases. Kids watch monsters in cartoons and learn about "bad guys" and "villains" on TV and movies. Inside us, fear is both a shadow and a friend we always carry around.

It protects us, but can also control us.

And it shuts us down, constricts us. Fear, or tension, constricts every part of our body, head to toes, lungs to saliva. People who are chronically in fear have dry mouths. Dry eyes. Dry skin. They always feel cold because they don't have much heat in their fingers or toes. They say they're "freezing" and are always reaching for a sweater or scarf.

When you begin to connect to your breath and start to tell yourself that you're safe and all is well, your body chemistry changes. You warm up—literally. Your energy starts to flow. Sometimes when people are stuck in fear, I have them clench their fists really tight—clench, clench, and keep clenching, even as they breathe. Eventually, they come to understand that this is how they are holding themselves all the time.

I ask them to keep clenching their hands. After a while, I tell them to let go. "Wow, this is amazing!" they say. It's a new sensation, different and wonderful at the same time. But they aren't really sure what to do with this new feeling. You could try this now—clench your fists, arms, legs, and toes really hard. Hold your whole body in that tight, tight way. Don't let go. Go even tighter.

Now release and breathe. Notice how that feels.

Helping clients feel safe and comfortable with a rush of energy and flow is important because if they've been clenching and fearful their whole life, and holding their body in a tight and constricted way, they may try to stop this flow. They probably saw their mom hold herself that way. They saw their dad hold himself that way. Fear feels familiar.

And if they aren't sensing their old fear, it seems like something is missing. They don't understand there's a whole other way to live.

And be.

And breathe.

This is a huge and very wonderful "a-ha" moment for lots of my clients.

Feeling relaxed, warm, and open, their energy is suddenly moving and flowing. And best of all, they didn't have to take a pill or have a drink to get there.

Now I bet you're wondering if this could happen for you. It can.

That's where I'm heading.

We all have this potential, I promise you. Because when you let go of fear, there's only one sensation left.

LOVE.

Love is what you have when you don't have fear.

When people begin connecting their breath and experience this delicious flow of energy, they want to have more of it. As they do the work, releasing fear, they begin to experience an even deeper and more constant kind of love.

Unconditional self-love.

Some of you may be surrounded by unconditional love for yourself already. Others may feel self-love some of the time, maybe just a random hour a week. But breathwork could get you there all of the time. It could take you to a place where you know your worth and your power. And where you feel safe.

When you love yourself fully, you do not need others to "make" you feel worthy. You are worthy already! You do not need to do anything or change anything.

Self-love is the foundation and the base from which we build all of our relationships. It has a profound effect on your life and the lives of the people around you. It could lead you to understanding love and having a more love-filled, love-centric, and loving life. That's a lot of love!

When I first started breathwork, I had no idea what unconditional self-love was or what it felt like; I certainly didn't know its importance or how to cultivate it. Breathwork helped me get past the stories that kept me from self-love. I connected to my strength and courage. It could do that for you too.

Self-love is the magic ingredient in happy relationships of all kinds. When you become aware that you are your own source of flowing energy and acceptance, the holes in your life and holes in your heart start to fill up.

How do you learn to love yourself?

It starts with listening.

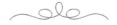

When you let go of fear, there's

only one sensation left. LOVE.

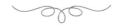

Love, Sex, and Relationships

My husband and I had things to work out when I started breathwork. He had married a woman who was afraid to be fully vulnerable and who often went into code-red. Breathwork began to change me. Don't get me wrong, I think he likes the real me a lot more. But it took some adjustment.

He was used to being with a partner who wasn't fully present and truly living in the moment. People who can't breathe and feel a deep connection to themselves also have trouble connecting to anybody else. It's hard for them to show up fully in a relationship. If you have tight, constrictive breaths, it takes much longer to let go, to be present, and to have an open and flowing connection with another person—and that goes for your sex life too.

And without feeling open and flowing, it is much harder to have a loose and juicy love life, as I mentioned in the last chapter. It's not that good sex is impossible without breathwork, or connected breathing, it's just that it helps you find that juicy place faster. You don't have the same walls and defenses and fear, because you are constantly releasing. You're not living in a bubble fortress that your partner has to work through to get you to that juicy place.

I mean, isn't that what foreplay is? You are being opened up. Your defenses and tightness are being worked out and released. A lot of times, one partner is literally helping the other partner get present, get open and loose, so that sex is enjoyable. If you have a breathwork routine, you don't need as much time for all that, for releasing and loosening up. You are not so clogged up in the first place, so you have more time for fun and play. And then, foreplay is just for the fun of it!

Self-love is an essential piece of this. If you love yourself, first and foremost, you are more relaxed. You are not existing in fight-or-flight mode. You are living with love—both love for yourself and love for others. In that open and flowing state, when you are breathing, there is a deeper trust and connection between you and your partner; there is a powerful oneness that transcends the physical connection and opens you to a more emotional and spiritual experience.

Besides better sex, the other thing breathwork gave my marriage was trust. I trusted myself and my husband more, and let go of fears that I was not enough. I let go of what I thought relationships were "supposed" to look like.

It's amazing how many people hold onto really conventional views about love and relationships, things that just don't make sense. Lots of them seem out of date—like that women should cook or men should work. One of these conventional beliefs is the idea that couples shouldn't spend too much time apart. Time apart raises fear. It seems threatening. With breathwork, I've learned the importance of spending time alone, learning about myself, and doing things for myself that make my heart sing. Before that, I felt guilty about alone-time. My family didn't understand why I wanted to go off by myself or "let" my husband have adventures of his own.

Why shouldn't he have his time too—to go diving and go skiing with our sons, or whatever he wants, whatever gives him joy? To me, getting to be alone and doing what brings you joy is part of relationship maintenance.

Otherwise, you are in *fear*, not love.

When you're in love, you trust your partner and you trust yourself.

What's good for one is good for both.

Luckily for me, and kind of by accident, my husband started doing breathwork too. Early on when I was still having panic attacks, and my breathwork classes were an hour away, he started driving me. When he saw what a difference breathwork was making, he took a class too. As soon as he did, it was a chance for us to reconnect on a deeper level again.

How?

When you get really present and you clear away the clutter, you can see beauty again. It's like your eyes open up and take in more. My husband and I began to see how much beauty there is between us, and how much there is in our marriage to savor. With that larger positive perspective, we were able to let the stories go—all the stuff that was ruffling feathers and making us irritated with each other.

Instead, we put our breath and awareness on all the good that was there. Our connection, our relationship, and our marriage began growing again. It's not like we don't ebb and flow. We still hit rough patches like anybody else. And breathing together has given us the trust and connection to know we will flow back again. We both understand that, and don't expect things to be perfect all the time.

We trust things will work out.

And that's a nice place to be.

Let's try a juicy breath exercise, just to get started. I want you to sit in a chair with your hands resting on your knees. Breathe in a full inhale while rocking your pelvis forward. Exhale while scooping your pelvis back and bringing your belly button to your spine.

Inhale. Arch your back. Exhale, and round your back. Repeat this ten times. And just close your eyes and notice how you feel—and if anything changes inside you. Do you feel any energy moving?

Choosing to Move On

Once you are more open, trusting, and flowing, you can see your relationships more clearly. Breathwork can be a catalyst for lots of changes in your life, and this isn't always easy. Sometimes that means you no longer feel like an energetic match with your partner. This is another way of saying you have grown apart. You are working on yourself and getting down to your authentic self. Your partner can choose to do some work too, and match your vibration, or maybe they don't. If they don't, you both may choose to move on.

As I mentioned in an earlier chapter, there is a way to separate as a couple that doesn't provoke bitterness, anger, and resentment. There really is! And I'm grateful to have witnessed this. In my practice, I've had clients let the drama and trauma go and move on in a gentle, harmonious way. One couple I know of decided to throw an "Untying the Knot" party. I loved this so much. Their child was happier and not forced to pit her parents against each other to gain control over where she'd live or which parent had "custody." An entirely new life was created that worked for each member of the family.

There's so much wisdom in this—using breathwork to release one another. A couple could continue to have a family relationship and a close friendship. They could continue to cheer each other on, even joyfully watch their partners move into new relationships, and grow, and deepen a connection with someone else.

How is that not a good thing? If you are truly living in the space of unconditional love, you want happiness for everyone.

To me, this is what real love is.

Self-love
is the
magic
ingredient
in happy
relationships
of all kinds.

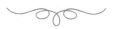

Self-Love and Breaking Unhealthy Patterns

Self-love doesn't just affect your relationships with other people, it also affects your relationship with yourself. When people don't feel worthy and deserving, they sometimes harm themselves or find ways to numb the feelings of unworthiness and not being loved; sometimes it's food, pills, drinking, shopping, smoking, or pot.

I have seen many clients find the power to confront these addictions when they were able to connect their breath, listen to themselves, clear out their inner stuff, and release and release. They discover the wellspring of love deep inside them.

Unconditional self-love doesn't happen overnight. Sometimes it is hard work. It's going into the trenches. It's walking your inner child around the block when you don't want to, or writing a letter to a family member, or confronting some stuff you don't like about yourself. We've all made mistakes. We've all managed to not live up to our highest ideals and best selves.

To get to a place of self-trust, self-acceptance, and self-love means a lot of forgiveness. It means letting go, letting go, and letting go some more. Exhale. Exhale. Exhale. You learn to forgo the stories in your head about what, why, how—and just be.

Just being present.

No stories.

No shame.

Learning to just be present—and having faith in what's inside you now, not yesterday, or twenty years ago, but right now—is a form of unconditional love.

That's not to say it has to be hard, or take a long time. Sometimes with smoking addictions, I've helped people kick their habit in a few sessions. They learn to take a connected breath every time they want a cigarette.

The urge to smoke is the urge to breathe. Right? Once the nicotine piece of it is gone, I show them how to take "breath breaks" instead of cigarette breaks, which gives them the same calming effect.

Same with pot addiction. Some people come to my practice because they are addicted to cannabis and can't imagine that anything else could calm them. Then they have some breath sessions and they realize *there is something better*. And it's cheaper. Air is free!

An Exercise in Self-Love

In my classes and breathwork sessions, sometimes I give clients a little homework to get them started on the path to self-love. I'll ask them to find a picture of themselves as a child and put it on their nightstand. You could start this way too. Put a picture of you as a baby or child by your bed. Look at it in the morning and every night before you go to sleep—and send that child some love.

Rescuing Yourself

Self-love is the magic ingredient and special sauce that makes great transformations possible in life. If I hadn't experienced it for myself, and seen what self-love has done for my clients, I wouldn't be so passionate about this.

Here's the basic message, loud and clear:
NOBODY NEEDS TO RESCUE YOU.
YOU CAN RESCUE YOURSELF.

When you connect to your breath you go from victim to hero.

You feel more courageous, because you believe in yourself.

Breathwork helps quiet and heal all the things you've heard that left you feeling unworthy, or the voices that said you were unlovable or wrong. *Don't wear your hair that way. Don't wear those glasses. You're getting fat.*

Sometimes it means going overboard a little. When clients first get the hang of trusting and loving themselves, I see them become very vigilant in their own defense. In the beginning, they may overdo it. They take very strong stands and want to make sure nobody messes with them again! It's actually really rewarding to see, because it's coming from such a strong place. Eventually they figure out they don't need to fight so much. They create better boundaries. They relax. They see they don't want or need to engage with so much drama and trauma.

Loving yourself can mean being quieter, more trusting, more patient. When you love yourself, you don't want to drag yourself through all those thorn bushes.

Other things happen, like once you have spent time in a clearer space, connected to yourself, you don't really want to be around negative people or be treated badly anymore.

You don't want to eat poorly.

You don't want to be drunk or hungover.

You don't want to get numb on drugs.

Once you get a taste of how it feels to love yourself, you don't want to go back. You become your own best friend. You pay more attention to yourself. You are kinder to yourself and silence the inner critic. The inner critic goes to the back seat.

You listen to your heart.

You keep yourself in the flow.

Once you love yourself unconditionally, you have the courage to make some really big changes in your life. You know things might get hard. You know the future is uncertain. And, at the same time, you know that whatever comes up in your life, you are stronger, more solid, more resilient.

Resilience is what the next chapter is about.

CHAPTER 7

LEAPING INTO THE UNKNOWN

Taking risks, speaking your mind, making big leaps—or just coping with tough stuff that is part of life—requires strength and courage. It requires something else too: resiliency. Losses and disappointments in life can be crushing if you don't have a way to process them and move on.

Resiliency means you can bounce back. As the Dalai Lama would say, you become like bamboo in the wind. Hurricanes, typhoons, all kinds of storms can flatten bamboo. And the next day, bamboo stands straight again.

Setbacks were crushing for me before I began breathwork. I was rigid and, instead of bouncing back from feeling bad, those difficult feelings stayed around inside me and kept me down. It was like I carried a playlist of songs inside me that left me feeling weak and unable to cope. My breath was tight and shallow.

One of the glories of breathwork was how it changed all that. Breathwork gave me the gift of resilience. I became flexible and less reactive. I was able to go with the flow. For the first time, I felt strong and courageous, like I could cope with anything or breathe with it and find answers.

The change in me was pretty drastic. I went from being a nervous and high-strung perfectionist who was always worried about melting down to being a mellower woman who could bounce back—and keep bouncing.

Sure, I still have setbacks and challenging feelings, just like anybody does. But now, they don't keep me down.

What comes first: courage or resilience? To me, they are inseparable, along with trust and feeling safe. These qualities are like the roots and branches of the same tree. They bring you balance and confidence. And they give you the power to stand up for yourself, to speak your mind.

When you have courage, trust, and resilience, your life changes. Because the way you live and love changes. Suddenly you can take on more. You can make bigger decisions, even decide to change your life completely. You have the strength to be true to yourself. And that means you take bigger leaps.

That Calm and Peace is You

A psychotherapist who's a friend of mine once asked if I could help her with a patient who was having anxiety attacks. The teenager was a graduating senior who had been accepted to college when her panic attacks began. Most kids are stressed by the thought of moving away from home for the first time. But this girl was struggling with something more. Sometimes, she was so overcome by anxiety and panic that her worried parents had driven her to the ER.

Her parents were extremely anxious themselves. And understandably so. Two years before, their older daughter had died by suicide—a sudden event they were still trying to process. Now, with another daughter in distress, they were going to do whatever it took to keep her safe.

The therapist hoped breathwork could give her patient more resilience, the tools to calm herself down and cope better. The therapist also thought breathwork could get to the root of the girl's anxiety faster. The months were passing and the girl's departure for college was approaching.

I was asked to come to my friend's office at first, to work with her patient in a familiar setting. The first session, I invited her to try laying down on a sofa in the therapist's office while I sat on the floor next to her, to breathe with her. Every five seconds or so, she'd nervously sit up and look around. She just didn't trust the process or trust me—yet.

After three sessions, she began to feel more comfortable and began coming alone to my office. We started making progress pretty quickly after that. In our first private session, she spoke about her older sister, how much she missed her, how sad she felt sometimes. The next session, she admitted she felt incredibly guilty. Suicide can leave overwhelming sorrow in its wake—pain that takes different forms. Guilt is one.

She used to fight a lot with her sister, she confessed. Not understanding anything about her sister's depression, she teased her a lot. They'd been rivals for so long, all their lives, really, that the girl hadn't been able to see her sister as anything but a pain.

Now she was left grappling with a lot of terrible feelings. Her mind raced with regrets, and stories about how things could have been different. She even worried she had been responsible for her sister's depression.

"I should have been nicer to her," she said. "I should have been a better sister. Maybe she's gone because of me."

At the beginning of the next session, before we started breathing, something she said really hit me.

"Sometimes I just feel like diving in the water and never coming up again."

She was fantasizing about her own death.

I invited her to close her eyes, breathe for a minute, and walk into that water—to imagine herself wading into the surf.

"What's happening now?" I asked.

"The waves are crashing over my head."

"Are you under the water?"

She nodded.

"What's happening now?" I asked.

"It's so calm."

I waited a little bit. "And now, what's happening now?"

"I'm kinda floating down, all the way to the bottom," she said. "I'm going to the bottom of the sea, to the ocean floor."

"What's it like?"

Her face looked so young suddenly, and sweet. She had connected her breath. "Wow, I feel okay down here. It's really nice. I feel peaceful."

"Can you look above you, at the surface," I asked, "where the waves are breaking?"

"Yes."

"But it's calm and peaceful where you are, right?"

"Right."

"That's you. That calm and peace is in you," I said. "That's your peaceful center. Stay there for a few more breaths. Stay there as long as you want. You have the superpower here to breathe underwater. And to connect to the calm energy flowing through you."

She was silent, just breathing.

"That feeling is allowed to be with you all the time," I went on. "That's yours, and comes from deep inside. Wherever you are, wherever you go, you are allowed to be there and feel peaceful."

Things changed for her after that. It was a really powerful session and a turning point. She was able to see a few things differently. It reset her. She realized it was okay for her to be peaceful, and okay to move forward, to let go, forgive herself, and live her own life. She broke through something that could have affected her for her whole life.

She became stronger each session. Each time I saw her, more pain was scrubbed away. More light was coming from her. She was shining—all on her own. Before that, her mind had been trying to keep her from shining. She thought it was not okay to live if her sister could not.

And she knew now she had a peaceful place to go, no matter what came up. She had tools to get her there. If the waves on the surface felt rough and were crashing around her, she'd be able to find that place of peace—where she could find the love, wisdom, and strength to handle what was arising—and to relax and let it go.

After nine months of breathwork, she was ready to go to college.

I knew it and she knew it. So, we came up with coping strategies. We decided if she felt uncomfortable breathing in her dorm room with a roommate nearby, she could do her connected breathing in a park nearby. Or she could do it at the beginning of a class, quietly sitting in her classroom chair.

Breathwork could not erase the tragedy of her family's devastating loss. But it gave her the tools to bounce back. She found her natural resilience. She checked in with me once or twice after she moved into her dorm, to say that things were going well. Recently, I heard from her parents that she had graduated.

I can make a pretty good guess that breathwork, and what she learned about herself, didn't just get this young woman through college, it awakened a force inside her.

And now she will always be awake. It will continue to make a difference for the rest of her life.

What kind of difference?

It could change the way she loves, the way she lives. It could change the way she eats, because she'll be more sensitive and conscious about it. She may want to make sure her children have a more peaceful birth. She may raise them in a different way, with more trust and love. Grandparent in a fun way. And when she comes to the end of her life, she may have a very different last breath.

Without fear.

This young woman had something inside her: a strong spirit and a way to connect to it. Reconnecting to her spirit, time and time again with a connected breath, would keep her resilient, trusting, and unconditionally loving to herself and others. And whatever she faced, she'd know there was a way to feel safe.

We Are All Resilient

Some people seem born with natural resilience. The truth is, we are *all* born resilient. We all have the natural ability to handle anything—to adapt, cope, and bounce back. That's why, with the tools of breathwork, anybody could build an inner, bamboo-like structure that is strong enough to handle storms and giant waves, even hurricanes, with flexibility and grace.

Being fearful might feel like a natural state too. Fear could rise when we are faced with change, and it could be a health change, geographic change, or a relationship change. Any kind of change. Each of us has different things that trigger fear. What seems huge to you—an unimaginably scary thing—may seem like no big deal or even an exciting adventure to somebody else.

It doesn't have to be as serious as a health issue, or the grief and guilt of a sibling's suicide. It could be anything at all. Anything that gives you that pinch or stab of panic and fear or anxiousness.

You've put your house on the market.

Your boss offers you a promotion.

You find out you're expecting twins.

Breathwork doesn't treat these situations any differently, because the basic condition is the same. You feel uncomfortable and not in control. Your world seems upside down. You can't catch your breath. The way toward peace of mind is the same. It's just a matter of learning to connect your breath seamlessly, where you begin to relax your body and focus on connecting the inhale and exhale. After that, you are able to quickly tap into your deepest and strongest self, where you feel safe and steady. The more time you spend in that place, and the more you forgive and love yourself, the stronger and quieter and larger that place inside you becomes.

Eventually, it becomes an internal structure that supports you and keeps you steady. What is that structure made of?

Self-acceptance.

Self-forgiveness.

Unconditional self-love.

Each time you connect your breath, you return to that place. The rhythm of your inhale and exhale alone will bring you back to balance. Connecting your breath will transform your fear into excitement.

And in time, once you have practiced experiencing your biggest feelings without pushing them away, you will find, in the midst of them, your own inner calm and strength. This will have enormous significance on everything you do. Because you won't be living in fear anymore. Your actions won't be driven by fear.

You will be up for whatever life is presenting you. And that's a game changer. Life is full of surprises—it's a wild ride with twists and turns—and it's an easier and more joyful ride when you take your breath with you.

We are all born resilient.

Facing Your Feelings Makes You Stronger

Sometimes in my group classes and retreats, I ask students to try to remember something that happened recently that stirred them up, that left them feeling uneasy or unsettled. Something that gave them a little pinch of fear or anxiety. I'd like you try this.

Just think of something small that caused feelings to arise, a faint unsettled feeling that isn't overwhelming. Something that mildly annoyed or irritated you, like someone cutting you off in traffic or a friend standing you up for your lunch date.

If you start with that small uncomfortable sensation and feel it fully, and practice connecting your breath and breathing with it, then you will begin to practice one of the essentials of breathwork. You will learn how to be more attuned to sensations inside yourself. You will not have to run from them. You will begin to breathe with them as they are happening and not have to stuff them down.

Take a minute now to describe the sensation you feel when you re-experience that mildly irritating situation.

Is the sensation light or heavy?

Smooth or rough?

Sharp or dull?

Hot or cold?

Keep breathing while thinking of your new description of the sensation—not the label (sad or mad)—without trying to change it. Really experience the *sensation*. Don't make it go away. Then, pay attention to what happens with the sensation as you connect your breath. Continue to pay attention to it. Feel the edges of it. The space around it.

Does the sensation stay the same or change?

As you practice focusing on the sensation, identifying it and feeling it, you will begin to notice that it dissipates. Sometimes, it just suddenly vanishes—poof! This is what happens in the letting-go process. You are releasing stuck energy. Releasing and releasing. Once you learn how to do that, you can try tougher stuff.

Soon enough, the bigger stuff doesn't seem so scary either. You realize you can ride those waves too.

Ride
the waves
with a
big smile.

Taking Those Leaps

Making life-changing decisions is challenging for almost anybody. Heading to college, breaking up with a partner, changing jobs, buying a house, even buying a new car. Breathwork helps us learn to take the magic slide from our head to our heart. We begin to trust our inner wisdom and guidance, and listen when our heart speaks. We take a leap toward our own desires.

I always took big leaps before I started breathwork. I was the kind of person who made up her mind to do something, or be something, and just did it. I wasn't afraid of the leap itself, but I was always fearful of upsetting the people I love. I was worried about what they would think, or that I wouldn't measure up to their expectations.

I vividly remember my epiphany about wanting to become a breathworker. I felt it in my heart, even though I had already invested years into my career as a photojournalist. This created a dilemma for me. My heart wasn't in sync with my head. In my head, I thought breathwork was supposed to be a healing practice that kept me from going code-red. In my heart, I knew it was my passion—and my new profession.

I couldn't stop thinking about teaching breathwork and helping people learn all the things I was learning. It felt right deep down. The feeling was strong. And whenever I connected my breath and thought about becoming a breathworker, things felt very clear to me. Suddenly, I knew it was my calling.

This wasn't obvious to anybody but me. My husband was really puzzled. I had gone to the trouble of getting a master's in journalism. Why change my profession now?

Even my parents and my kids were like … huh?

They didn't understand. And, as I've said, change is hard. And nobody likes it when change comes without any warning.

So, I stopped bringing up the subject with my family. I continued to know I was going to become a breathworker, and I was super excited about it, but I decided I didn't have to remind my family about it. They didn't grasp it yet. This went on between us for a while. I think my family was relieved. They were secretly hoping I'd changed my mind.

It felt lonely to be the only one who believed in my choices, though it was also affirmed to me, even more, how breathwork had made me stronger and more resilient. It gave me the tools to believe in myself. I realized something else: I needed to express confidence in my decision. The more composed and confident I was about it, the more supportive my family would be.

So, after a few months, I jumped in with both feet and told my husband I was sure. Breathwork was just something I needed to do. That's all there was to it! As soon as I did that, he could tell how strong I felt about the decision and how much it mattered to me. And he became really supportive.

Going through that experience has helped me with lots of clients who are grappling with the changes that come with breathwork. I have many clients—career politicians, attorneys, and teachers—who discover they want to do something radically different with their lives. They want to run a bed-and-breakfast in Vermont. Or they want to move to the beach. One client decided to become a chef in California.

I know how hard it can be to follow your heart's desire and be okay with being the only person who really understands it. Standing up for yourself and going against convention, and what everybody else thinks you should be doing, isn't easy. These kinds of decisions take courage and self-love. Once you connect with the powerful flow inside you, you can believe in yourself and go forward.

Breathwork opens up the channel between the deep, wise you and the one on the surface who is fighting the waves. Once you start listening to your heart, you'll hear some surprising things.

Your heart has its reasons.

And only you know what they are.

~ ∘ℓ∘ ~

Once you start listening to your heart, you'll hear some surprising things.

~ ∘ɤ∘ ~

My Emergency Toolkit

Clients call me at all times of the day, and sometimes at night, when they've been upset by something and are feeling a loss of control. "I don't know how to handle this," they say. Or, "I think I'm about to have a panic attack!" Just because you've gotten the hang of breathwork doesn't mean you are always 100 percent calm, cool, and collected.

Life has a way of giving out new challenges.

When I get a code-red SOS signal from a client, I have an answer ready, a checklist of things I have taught them to do.

These four things will work to get you calm and cool again, because I have turned to them myself, time and again, when I get off track.

Here is my Emergency Toolkit:

1

CONNECT YOUR BREATH

First things first. I ask clients in distress if they've taken twenty conscious connected diaphragmatic breaths—deep, from the belly to their chest. That's one surefire way to feel better very quickly. It works for me without fail. It lowers the cortisol and adrenaline in your bloodstream that makes you feel anxious and uncomfortable, leaving you feeling calmer. A conscious breath also puts you in a different part of your brain, your prefrontal cortex, a higher reasoning part. This helps you handle whatever is arising for you in a more centered and balanced way.

A great thing to try is to breathe in to the count of five, then exhale to the count of five. This is called coherent breathing. It calms and steadies the breath, which calms and steadies the mind.

2

DRINK WATER

Get hydrated, I tell them. My clients joke that my favorite drinking game involves only one beverage and it comes out of the faucet. So many people are drinking coffee or tea all day, and then wine at night. These are all dehydrating and take water out of you instead of putting it in. (There could be an H2O bar for people in crisis.) Being dehydrated is tough on the body, mind, and spirit. It makes your energy get stuck too. Drinking eight glasses of water a day will help you function optimally, especially if you are under stress. Also, when you do breathwork and all that respiration is giving you a great detox, your system needs more water than usual to help clear out the gunk your breath is releasing.

3

MOVE YOUR BODY

I ask about exercise. Have they moved their body today? If not, I have them do ten push-ups or ten sit-ups as I am talking with them. Get the blood flowing. Get the energy moving. Honestly, that may be all they need to change their state of mind and give them the ability to cope. Daily exercise is key to maintaining flow.

Another fun exercise is to stand up and think about something that makes you angry. Once the anger rises in you, start wiggling your whole body. Are you still mad? Pretty funny, isn't it? The mind lets go of anger as soon as it's moving.

4

GO OUTSIDE IN NATURE

They don't call it the "great" outdoors for nothing. Go outside, get into nature, feel the sky over your head. And be sure to keep breathing. Being in nature will change your perspective almost instantly. You hear birds chirping. You feel your feet on the ground. You feel the wind and sun on your face. You watch the leaves dancing in the trees. You can feel your own breath coming in and out.

Suddenly, you are present. The stories that were swirling inside your mind fade away. Whatever was stressing you out will suddenly feel small and manageable. When you connect with nature, serotonin, a chemical that regulates mood, is released in the brain, giving you a feeling of peace and emotional ease.

Even if you are at the office, there are plenty of ways to dig into my Emergency Toolkit before an important work call or meeting. It makes you more responsive and less reactive. (One of my clients likes to do push-ups against her office wall after she takes a walk around the block.) If you are facing a stressful family event, give yourself a little extra time to breathe, hydrate, exercise, and take a walk outside beforehand, and I promise you will feel kinder, more patient, and compassionate.

And if you are hit with a sudden unexpected blow, upset, or surprise, and you feel your breath getting shallow and constricted, you can turn to this list and find that everything becomes more manageable. It's probably not a bad idea to put a little note over your computer that says:

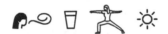

CONNECT YOUR BREATH.

DRINK WATER.

MOVE YOUR BODY.

GO OUTSIDE IN NATURE.

And keep breathing!
Ahhhh ... this list has saved me so many times.

Upward Spiral

We are all naturally resilient and so strong. But sometimes we forget what delicate, sensitive beings we are. We are strong and capable, but we also need to be taken care of, the way you maintain a high-performance race car. We need to be gentle with ourselves, have regular tune-ups to stay balanced. We need our engines to be clear and clean. Breathwork is one way to keep yourself balanced and clear.

Everybody has different needs. Some of us need a rigorous daily breathwork practice. Others are okay with a short one. For me to stay unstuck and resilient, I need more maintenance than a weekly breath session and I'm not ashamed to say it.

I never get out of bed in the morning without consciously connecting my breath for at least ten minutes. That can mean the difference between a jagged, disconnected day and one with profound insights and peacefulness. It's really that powerful and a way to feel wiser and more grateful. Breathing connects us to something greater than ourselves. When I finish breathing, I get out of bed and drink water. I play with my dog. I do yoga and then take a shower and start my day in a clear way. This means I am less reactive. This means I am listening to myself and open and present and alive.

I am living with love.

And I have courage to follow my heart.

When you have that kind of courage—and you're living in a vibrant and open way—you are much more in tune with your physical and emotional self. And there's no question this creates a far healthier you. That's what the next chapter is about.

Breathing
connects
us to
something
greater
than
ourselves.

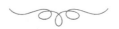

CHAPTER 8

THE HEALTHY COCKTAIL

When I'm asked about the power of breath to heal the body, I'm always a little reluctant to make claims that sound exaggerated. The rewards of a breathwork practice are uniquely different for everyone. At the same time, I have to confess—wow!—I have seen miraculous transformations occur.

Helping people get healthier and feel stronger is one of the things I love about facilitating breathwork. Sometimes it happens so quickly, like the client who wanted to learn some coping strategies for the emotional stress in his life. He had a code-red lifestyle that was getting the best of him. He never mentioned chronic pain, or anything specific like that, he just wanted some help living a calmer, more peaceful lifestyle.

In a private session, I led him through the basics, introducing him to creating intention, toning, and connected breathing. As soon as we finished, he bolted upright with a puzzled look on his face.

"Where did it go?" he asked. He looked around my breathwork room as if something had been taken from him.

"Where did *what* go?" I asked.

"The pain in my back. I've had it for thirty years. And now it's gone!"

I guess he was so used to his back pain, he hadn't bothered to mention it to me before our session. Typically I would guide someone's breath into an area where there is constriction to help them release the stuck energy.

Imagine that.

Thirty years of back pain … gone in one session.

"So weird!" he kept saying. "Where did it go?"

I smiled. It was almost like he missed that old pain!

"Well," I replied, "when you do breathwork, you clear emotional pain and that could help you heal physical pain. Because they are connected, right?"

He nodded a little skeptically. Like so many of us in the West, he had been taught that somehow his body existed in a totally separate universe from his heart and mind and spirit. It's astonishing that we separate them.

"At some point you may figure out who or what the pain in your back was," I said. "And it may not really matter since you've already released it."

This kind of experience is common in my practice, so common I want to highlight this sentence in boldface type: **It's not unusual for someone to come to breathwork for one thing and discover other parts of their lives coming into balance.** Most of the time, their health will improve along with their emotional state. Sometimes, like my client with the thirty-year backache, they are totally mystified when changes appear. Eventually, they become used to these changes as things in their bodies and lives come into balance.

How does that happen?

Breath allows you to trust yourself more. It brings emotional resilience and joy. And once you feel more centered and grounded, there is a pretty strong ripple effect. Suddenly your relationships feel different, more alive. Suddenly you are able to face a big decision at work—or make changes in your career or relationship that are more authentic and vibrant.

The benefits of your new strength and balance continue to build on each other. As you release and let go, clearing yourself out, you become more awake. You become more conscious of what you eat, how you exercise, and what your body needs to thrive and feel good. One of the reasons I don't make big overblown statements about the way breathwork improves our health is that breathwork isn't the only thing that produces these miraculous results.

Breath allows you to trust yourself more.

You are. That improved health comes with the awareness you develop as you do the work, as you face things, and as you feel more. It comes naturally, because you want to take better care of yourself, treat yourself better, the way you'd treat somebody you love.

Holistic Healing

How could the mind and body be separate? If you think about it for more than a second, it makes no sense. The human being is a whole being, a living and breathing network. Nothing about us is separate.

Anything that affects one part of you will have an effect on the whole being. When we experience emotional pain, how do we know?

We feel tight.

We feel burning.

We feel queasy—or tired.

Tears stream down our faces.

Our bodies are always responding. And our bodies take the impact of the feelings we don't want to face or feel. Anxiety and stress, even small amounts, make our hearts beat faster, our blood pressure rise, and could cause our brains to release chemicals that make us feel jumpy and jittery, which is why people under stress might find it hard to relax, concentrate, or sleep through the night.

Some of the old Western attitudes about the physical body being a separate entity—not connected to emotions or spirit—are fading away. Increasingly, I am seeing more openness to a larger view. The work of doctors like Deepak Chopra, Andrew Weil, Christiane Northrup, and Dean Ornish have introduced ways we can boost healing and well-being with holistic approaches. And over the last decade, there are more and more studies showing the health benefits of meditative practices like breathwork and mindfulness.

Chronic fear, or all the various labels we give it—stress, tension, anxiety, pressure, worry, nervousness, restlessness, irritation, anger, aggression, rage—creates an unhealthy imbalance in our bodies' intricate networks. Living the code-red lifestyle isn't just uncomfortable, it is toxic—worse for you than sugar.

Studies continue to back up what many of us instinctively know, that we are whole and human, each part of us connected, and feelings or stuck energy may create disease or what I call "dis-*ease*" in the body. Breathwork is effective in the treatment of a host of physical and emotional conditions, from enhancing joy, vitality, and sexual health to boosting the immune system, increasing lung capacity, improving digestion and heart health, helping in the treatment of addiction, and aiding fertility, pregnancy, and birth. Staying balanced, calm, and oxygenated can protect you from dis-*ease* and even help the brain from the effects of aging.

Change your breath.

Change your mind.

Change your life—and your health.

The Sound of Healing

A woman came to see me last year. She had a whole lot going on in her life. In her mid-forties, she was running a business as well as a household with a lot of kids, some with pretty challenging needs. She shouldered most of the responsibility for the family calendar, logistics, and getting the kids to lessons, practice, and school.

She had a pretty challenging health condition too. She was on several different medications for ulcerative colitis, or UC. It's a difficult condition to live with. The large intestine and rectum become inflamed and ulcerated, often resulting in severe cramping, chronic diarrhea, and fatigue. There is no easy cure for UC.

She arrived for her first session and I could see immediately that she was very tight from the stiff way she held her neck and shoulders. Even her facial muscles were rigid. Her smile was forced, polite, and automatic. She wasn't smiling so much as trying to smile.

As soon as we began working together, she took to breathwork right away. Just a couple sessions in, she was allowing her belly to become soft, deepening her inhale, and letting her body melt into the exhale. When big waves of emotion rose up, she connected her breath and was really getting good at riding them.

The weeks passed and she began changing before my eyes. I could literally *hear how breathwork was changing her*.

Her stomach made the loudest gurgling sounds as her belly opened up. At first, she apologized for the noisy symphony that was playing inside her. She felt self-conscious until I told her it was music to me.

She was letting go.

She was loosening up.

And it meant she was healing.

About four months into breathwork, her doctor began lowering the doses for some of her medications. She had no setbacks. A little later, she cut back a little more. Same thing. No setbacks. Her progress was slow and steady. She wasn't overly hopeful about a "miracle cure," but she wasn't going to rule out the possibility either. She's that kind of person. Careful, serious, responsible.

So, I had to ask her a question, one I truly had no idea how she'd answer: "What brings you the most joy?"

"Joy?" she asked.

It seemed like a new concept to her.

"What could you imagine doing for yourself," I asked, "that would bring *you* the most joy?"

She thought for a second.

"Sometimes I dream about going to Maine by myself," she said. "Our family goes there in the summer but it's not like I get a chance to really unwind. I'm always looking after things—cooking and driving the kids and organizing our activities."

"What if you went there alone?" I asked.

A smile broke across her face.

"What would that look like?" I went on.

"I'd wake up whenever I was ready to wake up," she answered, allowing herself to imagine it. "And maybe I'd just walk along the rocky shoreline, experience the morning sunshine, eat whatever I want, play music I love, and cook my own dinner at night. It would be like my own retreat."

At her next session, we talked about it again. "What would it take to make that happen?" I asked.

"I don't see how it's possible."

"Sure it is!"

"Okay, walk me through the steps," she said.

"Well, telling yourself it is possible is the first step," I said. "You must be able to envision it to manifest it."

"Okay."

"Allow yourself to feel that it is already happening."

"Okay."

"Now what would that look like?" I asked.

"Well," she said, "I guess I'd bring in a sitter who can stay overnight and look after the kids. And I'd ask my friend to carpool them to school and back. And then, I guess I'd let them skip a few things—miss their music lessons on Friday and soccer practice on Saturday. I mean, what's the big deal? Right?"

She was laughing by now. It was so infectious, I had to join in. She was reminding me of me, back when I was a perfectionist mom trying to make sure no balls were thrown in the house.

"If I got a flight on Thursday and came home on Sunday," she said, "that would give me three nights and almost three days." Her eyes were shining as she worked out a few more details for herself.

Next time we met, her trip was all set—flights purchased. By then, she was almost entirely off any medications. And that alone strengthened her sense of liberation, freedom, and joy.

Her transformation after she returned from her "retreat" was something else. Her spirit was so vibrant and alive. She looked almost ten years younger! And she was on her way to more changes. She had started running again and found more ways to do things for herself. She said breathwork had given her the courage to make the changes to feel better and bring more joy to her life.

There are so many things to love about this wonderful woman's story. What I love most is her trust in herself and her own process. Each of us is different. Each of us needs different things. And what we need today may be different from what we needed five years ago or may need five months or five days from now. She asked herself what her spirit desired—what it needed to feed her, to bring her joy, spontaneity, peace, balance, and a juicier and more rewarding life. She envisioned it and manifested it.

Becoming healthier was just something that happened along the way.

She did that herself—with the power of breath.

Doctor, Heal Thyself

For the last two years, I've been asked by one of the nation's top health insurance and medical care companies to work with a ballroom of 900 doctors at an annual conference. The first time I did this, I figured I would give a short talk about the patient experience. What kind of environment is soothing and would enable patients to feel safe enough to breathe and to share? And I thought I'd talk with the doctors about how diaphragmatic breathing could really help patients with stomach ailments as well as respiratory issues.

If they knew more about breathwork, I reasoned, they'd be more likely to instruct patients on the benefits of a full, less constricted way to breathe. And I hoped that they'd feel more confident about referring patients to certified breathworkers.

But the questions they raised weren't about their patients; they were about the doctors themselves. They were all so stressed! One doctor was going through a double mastectomy and asked for breathwork advice. Another doctor had a nervous tic and wanted to know if breathwork could help.

Funny I hadn't been able to guess that before I went. Of course doctors are stressed! As they described their work schedules—early hours, lack of sleep, the pressure that went with their jobs—I started to see how much these hardworking and committed people on the frontlines of healthcare needed to give themselves more TLC before they could give it to their patients.

How can you care for your patient if you aren't able to care for yourself?

The next year, I started my talk with self-care. Right away, I could sense a different level of focus from the audience. I was sharing information they already knew, deep down, but desperately needed to hear again.

After giving them a breathwork session, I suggested they make the time, between seeing patients, to put a hand on their belly and another one on their chest, and take five to ten breaths. Breathe between office visits. Breathe while making rounds. Just inhale and exhale, I told them. Take a breath vacation between patients, even if you have to do it while walking down the hall. And I led them through this breath-break exercise that can help anybody, anytime, become clearer and more present.

Let's start with a big socially unacceptable yawn. Open your mouth wide and make sure the air coming in is a noisy inhale. Exhale the yawn with a noisy sigh. Inhale the noisy yawn and squeeze your eyes tight. Exhale with them squeezed tight.

Check to see if your eyes are tearing. When your eyes water, you have released the tension in them—a great thing for keeping your eyes relaxed and not strained. Now try a full-body yawn. Raise your hands above your head and stretch, bringing your arms down on the exhale. This is a great way to release and reset.

Even if a doctor has only a few seconds between patients, I suggested they stand outside the treatment room and take three calm, slow breaths in and out. Wiggling their toes inside their shoes would be helpful, then having a quick full-body shake out could provide an added bonus boost.

This way, they can be fresher and more present for their next patient, and their wisdom and intuition—something doctors rely on—will be much more present too.

After these exercises, I asked the doctors what else they were dealing with day-to-day. I kept hearing the same thing.

Headaches.

Doctors get a lot of headaches.

No surprise, people who tend to live in their head and shoulders will collect stuck energy (a.k.a. tension) there. So, I asked the doctors to breathe into their shoulders, and move them up with the inhale and back and around with the exhale, to really open them up. Our shoulders are often where we hold the tension and emotion in our bodies—and where we wind up with tightness and pain if we aren't expressing and feeling our feelings and emotions.

Doctors are trained to make clinical decisions. At the same time, their work tends to bring up a lot of emotions.

Along with their own, they are probably feeling their patients' emotions too.

As soon as they started breathing with me, some doctors started tearing and others were giggling. I just wanted to hug them all and thank them for trusting the process. It was amazing how much they changed in just twenty minutes of connected breathing, and from telling themselves it was okay to take off their armor—to feel their feelings, to release and let go.

I get excited by the thought that these wonderful doctors will take what they learned from breathwork and pass it along to their patients and families. And, most important, use it on themselves.

Staying Open, Staying Healthy

Fear closes us down. Connecting your breath moves you from fear to love, which is very powerful. And it is powerfully healing.

A daily breathwork practice is like having an apple a day.

And once you recognize the sensation of energy moving in your body, you'll start wanting to keep it moving, clear, and unstuck. When your energy gets stuck, you'll begin to develop your own techniques for getting it moving again. The Emergency Toolkit is something to always keep in mind. It can help you get your energy moving again. Drink water, breathe, move your body, and walk in nature. You may also want to look at other holistic practices that enhance breathwork.

Anything that gets energy moving.

Anything that helps you release and let go.

There are so many fantastic options—yoga, acupuncture, Reiki (or energy healing), myofascial release, foot reflexology, and massage, to name a few. Both mindfulness meditation and some forms of Zen sitting practices have a pronounced breathing component and, for some, conscious breathing is the central aspect. I've also recommended some clients try Buteyko, a technique that helps people with asthma or chronic respiratory conditions by teaching controlled breath exercises.

Once your energy is moving, you feel a greater sense of all-over wellness: Your world opens up, becomes bigger and deeper and wider. Your heart expands. You have the bandwidth to be kinder and more compassionate. You have a more generous approach to your family and friends—and to perfect strangers who suddenly don't seem like strangers.

Because nobody really is.

We are all part of a central lifeforce, a current of divine energy that pumps through the universe and pumps through all of us. Breathwork opens you up to this current and could take you to a new way of being. A new plane of existence, a new way to love. It creates spaciousness that allows for profound insights. It also opens up your adventurous and playful side where you are able to delight in the pleasure of your senses.

Telling
yourself
it is
possible
is the
first step.

CHAPTER 9

DEEPER STATES OF JUICY

We need to have fun. And I'm deeply serious. Having fun and feeling joyful opens us up. Fun and joy get our energy moving. We are quicker to laugh, quicker to let go, release, and move on. So, throw out that to-do list! Prioritize fun!

Fun is the way to bring more juiciness into your life.

Juicy, as in giddy and silly.

Juicy, like when the sweetness of life is dripping down your chin.

When we don't have joy and juiciness, we crave it and look all over for it, although it is inside us, deep down, all along. Sometimes we just forget how to get there.

There's one sure way, though.

Start breathing.

Breath is a big, beautiful, badass doorway to this joyful state of mind. Experiencing our breath is a road trip to where our magic is. You start feeling different. You'll start feeling looser, noodly, almost giddy.

If you go a little farther, you'll feel your natural state of peace and bliss. Some people say they feel more meditative and relaxed doing breathwork. Others say they have had mystical or spiritual experiences. But more often, people say breathwork gives them an almost palpable boost of energy and joy.

Breathwork takes us to our source—our deepest place—where our life force and spirit reside. Where our passion is. Where ecstasy lives. In that place, we are more spontaneous, courageous, and playful. We are more inquisitive, curious, and creative. These states of being are linked and feed each other.

My Own Juicy

Art has always been my passion. I loved art classes when I was little. I loved playing with colors. I thought I might be an artist when I grew up. Art is fun and a way to play and express myself. But when I was in high school and excitedly enrolled in a painting class, I was crushed when I was led to believe that I had no talent.

The art teacher liked only one kind of painting: realism. We were supposed to paint barns, flowers, landscapes, and people. I felt like I was not good enough when he critiqued my work.

Never once did he offer constructive, positive ideas, or even notice that my thing was color, color, and more color. He never mentioned that maybe I could try abstract painting so I could apply my passion in another way. Instead, I just felt I couldn't paint. And I shut down.

Over the years, I channeled that love of color into my photography, photojournalism, and my work in music video production. Honestly, I never gave painting another thought.

Then breathwork came along.

I began the clearing out and releasing process that goes with the practice, and started feeling more courageous and more creative.

Over time, I really changed.

I was clearer.

And one of the things that got cleared away was that art teacher—and his criticism. Suddenly I had a deep, loud urge to bring more color into my life. I wanted to paint! And I wanted to find a teacher who was open to me playing with color and would encourage me, instead of giving me two million rules.

I wanted no rules at all.

I just wanted to have fun!

That new teacher appeared. *Hallelujah!* Now I can't stop painting. It pours out of me. Each canvas is an exploration for me, a chance to explore with color, movement, light, and energy. I put music in my ears and just start moving and let my energy pour out. I just get in the zone and start flowing, responding to what is happening on the canvas with another color, another shape, and I start moving my paintbrush.

My paintings are super-energetic. To me, they become a visual breath session and can shift energy, get flow moving. Not just in me, but in the people who see them and spend time with them.

Getting in the Zone

You never know where breathwork will take you. Any time your inner burdens are lifted, and you are freer and more open, surprises await. When you stop getting caught up in pleasing other people—and judging yourself—you find you have a lot more energy to pursue your passions. Even passions you never knew you had.

Breathwork gets almost everyone into the zone, whether it's painting, writing, playing soccer, playing guitar, gardening, or all the above.

In my group classes, people who said they never could sing, all of a sudden start getting really into the toning part of breathwork and they're like, "Wow. I want to go explore that, and take some singing lessons!"

Lots of people say they've always wanted to draw or play the piano but decided, at some early point in their lives, that they had no talent. I tell them my story about returning to painting. What I've seen over the years is that if you have passion and energy, you can make it happen.

One client of mine knew nothing about drawing, but always wanted to learn, so she signed up for lessons. When she started—and I'm not kidding—all she could draw was stick figures. Her sketches were really primitive. But she had bigger goals in mind. She was determined to master pencil drawing.

Six or seven years later, her drawings are now incredible. She didn't let herself get discouraged or listen to dismissive comments. She stayed on course and headed toward her goal. It took time, practice, and commitment, and without all the judgment and outside pressure, the journey was a joyful experience.

That's the other unexpected thing. How easy hard work can be if you are connected to your spirit. Without all the doubts and self-judgment in your head, you can just keep doing it, learning more, and chipping away at it. This is what expertise in anything requires.

Does this mean your inner critic never knocks at the door?

Being
comfortable
starts
with
feeling
safe.

Fear has a way of showing up, no matter who you are. Sometimes when I'm painting—even when I'm really in the zone, and flowing and excited—I'll do something with my brush and suddenly the canvas looks terrible. Like I've ruined the whole thing.

For a fleeting moment, my body tightens and I start criticizing myself, like, "Really? Why did I do that?"

Then I catch myself and start breathing to see if I can change the sensation. Sometimes it takes a little more than a few connected breaths and I dig around in my Emergency Toolkit. I drink water. I walk outside to clear my head. When I come back inside, I put my headphones back on and get music in my ears, pick up a brush, and just go to town again.

Right away, I'm giggling to myself. Not just because I'm joyful and creative again, but because I'm laughing at myself and my process. It's so funny how fast and simple it is to return to a state of greater awareness. It's easy, *so easy*.

I joke to myself, "What's the big deal? Please! There are no mistakes—right? And besides, I can paint over that funky brushstroke. I got this!"

Painting, in that way, has taught me a lot. It's like I'm taking my own one-woman workshop in letting go and letting flow. Creative work for my clients frequently gives them these same realizations and lessons. Whether they are singing, cooking, or gardening, it is another way of allowing themselves to enter into a joyful zone, and of learning to be courageous and comfortable to keep leaping into the unknown.

You learn to have *trust*.

And that's how you get in the flow again. That juicy flow.

Joyful Fun Sex

Sex! You were probably wondering about that. Yes, it is definitely one of the things that could change with breathwork. It takes so much courage to become comfortable and relaxed and loose enough to get to the deeper state of juicy. You have to be able to ask for pleasure, say what you need—and make noise.

Half the pleasure could come from the sounds you make!

They allow you to open up even more.

There's even a book about that, *Urban Tantra: Sacred Sex for the Twenty-First Century* by Barbara Carrellas, who discovered that sexual sounds gave her a connection to the ultimate spiritual experience.

Make noise!

And more noise!

Sure, it's true there could be spiritual revelations while connecting your breath while having sex, as Carrellas says. But most of my clients don't come to me with questions about finding God. When it comes to sex, they are just having trouble asking for what they need or want. They are looking for courage.

Being comfortable starts with feeling safe. Courage starts with self-love. When you have safety and self-love, you are capable of expressing your needs and wants. So much is possible when you are in this juicy flow.

So, how could you start on the road to feeling safe and trusting?

Feeling safe starts with experimenting with *yourself*. What feels good to you? When and where are you able to go out of your comfort zone? Self-pleasure is the beginning of the love story—with yourself and possibly with a partner.

Ask yourself some questions. What type of touch do you like and where do you like it? How much light do you like in the room, or do you like candles flickering? What smells do you like? What music gets you in the groove? How do you want your sheets to feel—silky smooth or cottony soft? Do you like the taste of rich chocolate or juicy mango?

Once you feel safe and playful, you are more open to new experiences with yourself or with a partner. Maybe you have a partner and you've been together a long time and gotten into some dull sex grooves. Breathwork can bring the courage to try new things. You can express your needs—and some wild fantasies, why not?—without fear you are going to crumble.

And if you are single, and looking for romance, you will feel a lot less fearful about dating and meeting new people.

I know I sound like a broken record, but it all starts with feeling safe and loving yourself. These two things bring you the courage to experiment, to be spontaneous and creative. And by being in the juicy flow, acting on those impulses, and allowing yourself to be present and playful, you will feel new energy and have even more new ideas.

So much is possible
when you are
in this juicy flow.

One exercise I give clients who tell me they want to feel juicier is to try something I call "cuddle breathing." It's a simple and powerful way to create intimacy.

Here's how it goes:

Try resting with your partner in a quiet, cozy space and begin to breathe together. You could do this on a bed or sofa, lying side by side, spooning, or one person lying on the chest of the other. Connect your inhale and exhale while your partner does the same. Now start noticing everything you can about your partner: the heat of their body, the touch of their skin, how their belly moves while they are connecting their breath.

Being fully present with someone is very sexy. And breathing together in this way keeps you out of your head and in your body. If you want, you could try this exercise while lying on top of one another with your clothes on, so you both feel safe and not pressured.

Keep feeling each other's breath and body. Feel the rhythm of your breath and theirs, and try to coordinate them, so you are breathing at the same rhythm and you become one. This brings a sense of openness, freedom, and excitement. Sometimes that's all you need to reconnect, and feel juicier.

If that feels like too much, or one of you isn't comfortable with that level of physical contact, you could try putting your left hand on your partner's heart. Ask your partner to do the same and put their left hand on your heart. When you each have a hand on the other's heart, start breathing together while looking into each other's eyes.

This is a quick way to change the conversation between you and your partner. You are sharing heart energy and deeply connecting. You are opening up and doing something new.

It doesn't take much sometimes.
Just a shift of mood.
Some nice music.
Letting go. Releasing the old stories.

With your hands on each other's hearts, keep breathing. Feel the rhythm of their breath. Smell each other's scent. Feel each other's body moving. You can send your love to each other without words; just imagine yourself inhaling a white sparkling light into your heart and then exhaling it and sharing it with your partner's heart. You are sending love back and forth to each other. This can be every bit as intimate as full-on sex, just sharing heart energy in a quiet space together.

Or Try This—By Yourself

Some clients say they just can't feel pleasure anymore. It may have started when they didn't feel safe or feel trust. Maybe they've been in fear-mode for a long time, and the joyful part of them is shut down.

Being unable to feel pleasure means your energy is stuck. The body has a way of getting into grooves and habits in an effort to protect you and keep you safe.

It often doesn't take much to get into pleasure-mode again. It starts with beginning to experience pleasurable touch again—in a safe way.

Find a comfortable, cozy spot.

Roll up your sleeve and start breathing a long soft inhale and exhale.

Stroke your forearm, on the inside where you have more nerves and pleasure sensors. Start at your wrist and slowly work your way up your arm with an inhale, all the way above your elbow. Take your time. Take a minute to do this—and then reverse direction and stroke your arm all the way back to your wrist with an exhale.

Keep breathing, and keep moving your fingers slowly. If this makes you feel tight and constricted, breathe into the tightness while experiencing it. Then let it go. *Release, release.* Allow yourself this little bit of pleasure. Make it safe for yourself, and see if you can accept and trust this sensation.

Keep breathing, nice and slowly. Once you begin to get comfortable with pleasure on your arm, you will eventually begin to crave it elsewhere.

Where else do you crave it?

What interests you?

Start paying attention to what lights you up, what feels good. Pleasure is a wild scavenger hunt. Everyone is different. Discover your urges. You may want to take a warm bath and explore your body more.

Keep breathing.

I am safe.

I am enough.

Nothing else is really needed, you know. As you sit in that warm bath, remember you don't need anyone else to complete you—or bring you pleasure. Having a good physical relationship with your own body is enough. It really is.

The Road to Ecstasy

Bliss is only a breath away. Ecstasy can sound like an extreme and elaborate goal. If we load the word with too much expectation, it can seem unattainable, like reaching enlightenment.

It is much simpler than that. The word comes from "ex stasis" or being outside your usual state. It doesn't require exotic substances, great quantities of alcohol, or walking across hot coals.

For the journey, you need only two simple things. And you already have them inside you: trust and self-love. These give you the courage to ask for more in life.

- More epiphanies
- More adventures
- More pleasure

All of these are linked and continue to feed you. Each time you are joyful and creative, allowing yourself to let go, play, and laugh, it feeds other parts of your spirit. One creative act leads to other creative acts. So, for me, when I get stuck working on one painting, I'll start another one—or just start dancing. All the joyful energy inside us is nourishing to our minds, bodies, and spirits.

Ready to up your game? *Onward and upward!*

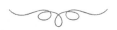

Bliss is only
a breath away.

CHAPTER 10

YOUR SHINING SPIRIT

Beyond emotional mastery is another doorway. Once you have learned to ride the waves, big and small, there's a passage to more growth. Whether you are a total beginner or you've been doing breathwork for a long time, the most astounding discovery is how much more there is still to experience. The doorways keep coming. Breath takes you to your authentic self again and again. Once you are connected to your deepest center and life force, you'll recognize pretty quickly that this place inside you is sacred. It generates a sacred feeling.

That is the feeling of your own shining spirit.

And that feeling is LOVE.

It's the kind of love that heals you.

And it's the kind of love that changes you.

This discovery is what floored me the most about breathwork, when I first started. I felt warm and safe, loved and cared for. I felt protected. Best of all, my spirit was so vibrant and alive, it was shining. The feeling and life force I experienced inside myself was big and connected to everything else alive, everything on Earth, and everything in heaven too. It was like I was hooked up to a huge energy field that was all-encompassing, universal, endless, and timeless. I didn't even know what to call it.

Spiritual awakening? *What is that?* Suddenly, I felt I wasn't alone in the universe; I wasn't separate from it. I was part of it, and that meant I had a team supporting me.

Some people call this Universal Love. Some call it God or Goddess, the Life Force, or the Divine. I think it's all that and more.

As a little girl and young woman, I never could have imagined having such a grand, all-encompassing feeling—and being comfortable with it or accepting it. Looking back now, I can see how disconnected I was. It was like I had been in a dark room and all of a sudden someone switched a light on. Breathwork didn't just help me connect with myself. It helped me see that I was connected to the world around me, and a higher power. I could see things clearly. My past no longer defined me. My entire future seemed open, and with each breath a chance for a totally fresh start. I could choose to parent differently. I could choose to live and love differently. I was able to let go of the stories and see things from a new perspective.

What healed me—and I could really feel it happening, the more I let go and released—was finding that wellspring of love within me.

It had been there all the time, my whole life, and I never knew it.

It wasn't just "love" in lowercase.

It was *LOVE.*

My life changed after that in so many ways. Mostly, the more time I spent breathing, the better and richer and deeper and truer my life became. I was becoming my authentic self, the person I was meant to be all along. There was no reason to look outside myself for a magic fix, mood lift, or safety. All the healing, wisdom, and guidance were already inside me. And as I began living in a connected way, listening to what my instincts and my heart were telling me, I began to hear my spirit. Experiencing breath was so powerful—and empowering.

As I got stronger and more courageous, I wondered, "What else is there?"

"What *else* have I been missing?"

A lot more.

SO MUCH MORE.

Even now, after years of teaching and training in breathwork, I feel that way. I still wonder what's coming next, what will unfold today, and what other mysteries and surprises are waiting for me. My sense of awe and wonder keeps growing. Divinity and magic can show up anywhere, at any time.

Every day is a surprise.

It all starts with one simple idea: You are divine energy.

Once you accept that, and tap into it, your life will change dramatically.

Beyond Emotional Mastery

When I was a baby, I could not fall asleep by myself. My mom would set me down in the crib and put her hand on my back until she thought I was fast asleep, then she'd crawl out of the room, sneaking out, hoping I didn't see her leave.

That's when I would start crying again. I'd cry my lungs out. I had terrible separation anxiety. I think it's because I lost a connection with my spirit or life force very early on. I was reaching out for external soothing and love. I needed to be very close to my parents to feel connected and safe again. Being alone in my crib at night didn't feel safe.

Quite often the things we experience as children, before we can even speak, stay with us into adulthood. When we breathe, emotions related to these early experiences and impressions can show up without a specific memory. When I started my own breathwork practice, I often sensed emotions welling up that didn't seem connected to an actual event.

What the heck was happening? Was my childhood that traumatic? While breathing, I would be overcome by strong waves of sadness, other times joy. These didn't seem to be "about" anything in particular; just a strong sensation that came without explanation. My breathworker taught me to really feel these feelings and breathe with them.

Once experienced, they were easy to release.

They were like clouds passing overhead, and drifting away.

Where did they come from?

Michael Brown's *The Presence Process: A Journey into Present Moment Awareness* offers explanations that are in sync with my own experiences of these fleeting "sensations" and also builds on what psychologists know about child development and early emotional imprinting.

Our emotional life begins in the womb. When we're in our mother's belly, we get vibrational imprints. These imprints are deeply suppressed and programmed into us, almost like genetic code. We can't really access them or remember them. These imprints explain why, sometimes, when you're breathing and something comes up, you begin crying for no apparent reason. There are no words or memories to attach to these sensations because they are things you experienced as an infant, perhaps even in the womb, before you had language and before you had concrete memories to draw on.

After you are born, and for your first seven years of life, most of your development is emotional. Sure, you are growing each day, and moving through the early developmental steps, but this is not happening consciously, the way we aren't conscious of our nails and hair growing. It is just happening.

Feelings are different, though. They are conscious. And during our first seven years, we learn what feelings are and attach words and experiences to them. People tell us what to call them and teach us to label them "good" or "bad."

This is how the socialization process works. This is how we learn how we are "supposed to react" to our own feelings—and how to react to the feelings of other people around us.

Most of us learn it's bad to cry.

We learn crying is noisy and disruptive.

We learn crying makes the people around us feel bad too.

We learn that only babies are allowed to do it.

As we grow up, we get better at suppressing our true feelings. This tends to make our parents and teachers really happy, and we are praised for making our feelings go away by tamping them down, pretending they aren't there. The Big People want us to grow up by learning to control our wellspring of feelings.

Between the ages of seven and fourteen, when we are in school, most of our growth is mental. We learn to think.

And then, from the ages fourteen to twenty-one, most of our growth is physical. We're back in our bodies; they change and grow quickly.

So, what kind of growth comes next?

Physically, there are lots of changes that come with aging, as we know. Intellectually, depending our work and lifestyle, there can be lots of growth as well. Unfortunately, though, for many people, there is little or no emotional growth for the rest of their lives. Emotionally, their seven-year-old is running the show. They reach an age of physical maturity and cognitive capability, but their emotional growth has stopped.

They live a largely reactive life.

A stressed and anxious life.

This is where breathwork comes in—and why it could feel so immediately powerful and effective. It facilitates the emotional growth our spirits have been waiting for. It's what we've desperately needed but society, and following the conventional paths, hasn't given us. Once you begin breathwork, you learn to ride the waves that come with emotional growth, and become stronger, calmer, and more courageous. You learn to feel your own feelings, experience them, and choose for yourself how to respond. This is emotional mastery and emotional maturity. You begin to experience your own energy and power.

Eventually, as you experience and release more and more, you no longer need to label your emotions. You are just present with them. You stop preferring them to be any other way. There is nothing to do but be with that energy.

With that emotional mastery comes renewed spirit. The child inside you—who was tamped down and taught to keep quiet—is now expressive and expansive. And the enlightened side of you, or your inner wisdom and intuition, makes room for that vibrant child. When we live from both our enlightened self and our vibrant child, we are in the flow.

When you are in the flow, you know.

What It Means to Be Spiritual

Just like the words "ecstasy" and "enlightenment" could seem loaded and difficult, the whole idea of embarking on a spiritual journey could intimidate people.

But guess what? You are already having one.

If you are reading, you are.

If you are breathing, you are.

You experience it every time you're in the zone with a perfect play in your favorite sport. You experience it when you are dancing, painting, gardening, cooking, or whenever you sense you're in the flow. A little kid on a soccer field can sometimes sense, before they even raise their foot to kick the ball, that they're about to make a goal. They get a massive high, even before the ball hits the net.

When you are in the flow, you know.

It's a sensation you have felt. It's something we all feel. It's spaciousness. It's ease. It's warm and big and calm. It could occur anywhere and anytime—a bus, a walk in nature, sitting in a coffee shop.

It's what we see in the eyes of the people we love, the animals we love, strangers across a room, friends, and family. In the eyes of others, we recognize ourselves. We are all one. This is how we are all connected. Behind the eyes in front of you is you in another form.

That is what I mean by spiritual.

And when you live in a fully connected way, you open like a flower. People are attracted to you because you have a different feeling about you; you are living fully, and expressing something that's authentic and true. There is a stillness about you, and a oneness, that keeps you calmer and wiser. You can stand in your own power. You make things happen with the intentions you create and manifest.

When you are consciously connected to your breath, anything is possible.

Ready to see what I'm talking about?

So far, you've learned how to connect your breath in a circular motion, by taking a diaphragmatic breath from your belly to your chest. And you've learned to relax with the sensations in your body.

Let's go a step farther, putting all the things you've learned together, and try a mini breathwork session on your own. An average breathwork session in my practice runs about one hour. For those just starting out, though, I suggest this first self-session last about five minutes. You'll want to build up slowly to something longer, or wait to see a breathwork coach for that.

Let's Put It All Together

Find a quiet place where you feel warm, safe, and undisturbed. Sit on a sofa or floor cushion. Bonus points if your head and body are both fully supported.

And let's talk about music. You don't have to do this in silence, unless that's what you want. You could choose a song or two to play for five minutes. It could be something instrumental, without voices or singing, that is uplifting and energetic but not too fast and not too slow. (If you are curious about my own playlists for breathwork, I share them and update them on my website, *experiencebreath.com*.)

Create an intention for this short session. Find words for the way you want to feel or what you want more of today. If you are feeling anxious, you could say, "I am calm." If you are feeling tired, you could say, "I am vibrant."

Put both your hands on your belly and begin to **breathe** into them.

On your **inhale**, your belly goes out. Watch your hands rise.

On your **exhale**, your belly goes back in.

If you've got that part down, and find belly-breathing comes naturally to you, move one of your hands to your chest or heart, and just keep one hand on your belly.

Begin taking full diaphragmatic breaths, in and out through your nose or mouth at your own pace, from your belly to chest. Seamlessly connect your inhale and exhale. Try not to pause between these. Check to see that your breath is a continuous loop of inhale and exhale.

Notice all the sensations that arise while you breathe. Make no effort to change these sensations or even judge them. Just let them happen. You may start to feel some tingly sensations, tightness, twitching, or swirling energy. If you feel lightheaded, slow your breathing down until that feeling passes. When it does, you could start to build your breath again.

On your next exhale, allow yourself to relax deeper into the support of the sofa. Let your body be heavy and fully relaxed. Keep melting and relaxing your body, as much as you can, while breathing fully. Sometimes it takes a while to let go of automatic or habitual body tension.

Soften your facial muscles, and even try to softly smile when something challenging comes up for you. This will begin to change your relationship to sensations.

If a sensation feels really uncomfortable or frustrating, you can have fun kicking and pounding your fists on the sofa and moving your head from side to side, toning *ahhhhh* as loudly as you can. This feels fantastic and really moves the energy inside us.

No judgments. No resistance. Just unconditionally love whatever is coming up for you. Allow it to happen. Allow it to come. Pay close attention to what arises. Be completely present with it. Don't try to resist, just allow it to be there, and then, just watch it drift away. At the end of your session, after five minutes, start to slow your breath down to its natural pace, in and out through the nose.

When you are ready to get up, go slowly. Your body has processed and released energy. It needs time to regroup. And when you are able to sit up or stand, take a moment to check in. How are you feeling? You could journal any thoughts or ideas that came up. Then, please, be sure to reach for a glass of water. When you do breathwork, you need to drink a lot of water. It's good to hydrate after breathing. Breathwork helps release the toxins in your body, and we need water to flush them out.

After your session, allow yourself quiet time to integrate.
  Sip some tea.
  Take a walk in nature.
  Look at something beautiful.
  Take a warm shower or soak in a tub.
  Just be.
  Just be *you*.
  And that alone is quite a miracle.

Next Steps

As you begin your breathwork journey, you'll probably experience many different sensations. Some are comfortable, some are uncomfortable. Whatever arises for you, as you breathe, or after you breathe, just know it will all be okay.

Things may be easier for you if you start with a certified breathwork coach. See if there is someone who holds classes or sees clients privately in your area. If there's a workshop, you might want to go. Check out my website for workshops and retreats and the International Breathwork Foundation website (ibfnetwork.com) to find a breathworker in your area.

Some people find that doing breathwork in tandem with talk therapy can be helpful with processing and integrating past experiences or current challenges. I have worked with several clients who said combining the two therapies together was life-changing.

We talked earlier about my Emergency Toolkit. As you do breathwork, this toolkit remains a critical component. It is reliable and simple and brings results. As you continue this journey, breathing, drinking water, exercising, and walking in nature will help you move the energy and feel clear, grounded, and balanced.

Some other things I recommend to my clients are:

Begin each day with at least **five minutes of breathing**.

Keep a journal to write your hopes and dreams. It could also be helpful to write about your breathwork experiences to help you process and integrate whatever bubbles up.

Think about what makes your vibrant child happy and **go do it**! Whether it's riding a bike, climbing a tree, baking a cake, or finger painting.

Spend time **imagining your heart's greatest desire**—and that you are already doing it. Writing a Broadway play, starting a company, jumping into a relationship, going on a trip—take a leap of faith.

High-Vibe Friends, High-Vibe Places

Once you do breathwork, you'll notice it shifts your relationships—with your partner, family members, and friends. Even if none of your loved ones are doing breathwork, your relationship with them will change because you are changing.

And when you grow, they may start to grow too.

Or, they might walk away.

Along those same lines, you will begin to attract, and be attracted to, other types of people, another set of friends and other kinds of relationships. I've seen this happen many times with clients. Once they are breathing, having emotional growth, and experiencing a more spacious and spiritual life, they will find themselves making new friends in their classes and retreats, or just sitting in a coffee shop or on a plane.

Once you're breathing and doing the work, getting juicier and deeper and more vibrant, you'll feel more alive, creative, connected to your authentic self. So, naturally you will gravitate to people who are connected to their juicy flow too.

You'll want to dance and sing and celebrate life!

A nice ripple effect happens next. Once two people who are on a similar spiritual journey meet and begin to share their experiences, they will learn more ways to grow from each other. They learn about other practices, other classes, other tools in addition to breathwork. There are so many paths that lead to the same shining place. I always encourage my clients to try other routes and different types of breathwork to keep growing and discovering.

When more enlightened people live in the world together, more healing can happen. There are amazing people everywhere, especially if you start looking for them. Seek them out. Support them, reassure them, let them know the wisdom and spirit they bring to the world make a difference. Every action affects everyone and everything.

When you start to radiate a sense of peace and happiness, friends and family around you might become curious. They may want to know what's up with you. And they may want to try some of what you've been trying. *They will see what you've gained and want some too.* This is one of the most beautiful ripples of breathwork, or any work on yourself. When you find your wisdom, this allows others to find theirs.

With breathwork you have a greater awareness of the world around you and your place in it. The clearer and better you feel inside, the clearer your relationship with the world becomes. You understand that we are all in this together, connected by energy and by each breath we take.

Not only are you creating and manifesting your own dreams, but you want to help create a better place for all of us to live. A calmer and more peaceful place. An environment that nurtures the spirit. This leads to even greater awareness—to people who are working with both their hearts and their heads—and creating environments where there's more consciousness, more conscious breathing, more conscious living and healing.

We are *all* on a spiritual journey.

Remind yourself of that every day.

Breath by breath, we can reconnect to something greater than ourselves, knowing something out there has our back. And knowing we are never alone.

Change your breath.

Change your life.

Change the world around you.

Your Journey

I created an intention at the beginning of this book, when we started this work together: *To help deepen your connection to your breath and yourself, to enhance your life in big beautiful ways, to encourage you to be brave and ride the waves of your emotions with a smile. To empower you on your own breath journey.*

I hope *Breath LOVE* has given you even more than that. Your life is yours alone to live and manifest. I hope I have helped you see what is possible, starting with emotional mastery and then continuing.

If you keep asking for more, you will get it.

A joyful life.

A juicier life.

Ecstasy and trust and love.

Connecting to your deepest self, your source or spirit, will be one of the greatest game-changers of your life. You are not alone. None of us is alone. This is one of the things you will come to understand. We are all connected and share a beautiful planet. Connecting to your own shining spirit will give you the strength to be more present and more vulnerable with people, something that facilitates deeper and richer relationships built on mutual trust. You'll experience a torrent of love, a waterfall, a gusher.

And you'll realize it is all coming from the same place. You.

LOVE—it is our life force and the spirit within us. It is the essential energy of life. It's what makes life worth living, what makes us want to wake up in the morning, excited to take on a challenge, to be surprised, to meet a new person, to hear a song. To dance our dance. Even when it feels hard, keep going. It will be worth it, I promise.

Your journey begins now.

Take a slow, deep breath and enjoy.

Your life is yours alone to live and manifest.

LOVE—
it is our
life force
and the
spirit
within us.

GRATITUDE

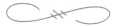

This book has been a dream of mine for a long time. A magical journey filled with LOVE and joy and breath. It wouldn't have been possible without the support of so many people. I am deeply thankful to those who have helped turn this dream into a reality.

First, I want to thank you—yes, YOU—for your willingness to open yourself up to the deeper possibilities of breathwork.

I am grateful for my breath teachers, Jessica Dibb, Judith Kravitz, Jim Morningstar, and Robert Winn—and for the teachers who taught them, Dr. Stanislav Grof, Leonard Orr, and Sondra Ray—for sharing your depth of knowledge, stunning insights, and love of breath. Your enthusiasm and wisdom are infectious and have deepened my own journey.

Next, I'd like to thank my incredible clients who inspire me every day and my loving community of fellow breathworkers for all their teachings and time. A special thank you to Alice, Kappy, Heather, Sandy, James, Ari, Terri, and my whole IBF family for your love and support.

Marie-Therese Maurice, for your countless hours of collaboration with me. Thank you, breath sister.

Deborah Norris, you are a wonderful friend and mentor. Thank you for believing in me and for creating with your loving family The Mindfulness Center in Bethesda, Maryland, a healing space where I have seen so many breathwork transformations.

Next, I want to express a river of gratitude for this book's Dream Team. I am in awe of their professionalism, sensitivity, patience, and playfulness:

Jodi Omear, there are no words! No words. Thank you for midwifing this book at all hours with me. Martha Sherrill, thank you for pouring your heart and soul into this project and helping me find the simplest way to say complicated things. Tammy Jones, thank you for your editing magic, wisdom, and humor. Elizabeth Casal, I'm grateful to you for making my dreams come true with the most beautiful book cover ever.

At Warren Publishing, I'd like to thank Mindy Kuhn, Amy Ashby, and Jen Hurvitz for believing in *Breath LOVE*. I am grateful for the way you've invested time and resources into this book and for your exciting plan to help me launch it to the moon. Tory Cowles, my amazing friend and awesome art teacher. I am so grateful you helped me get my painting mojo back! Your class has brought me deep healing. And I'm grateful for our merry band of classmates!

And there's Kenny, my close bud who got me to my first breath session. Did you know where that would lead? Thank you for starting me on this life-changing journey.

Wendy, Jessie, Carole, Najmieh, Charlotte, Maria, Missy Miss, Kay, Tracy, Leah, Tracy, Cleo, Debra, Ginny, Alice, Eve,

Nicola, Cheryl, Nora, Brenda, Mary, Melanie, Courtney, and so many others who all bring out my playful side. My life is fuller with you in it.

And now, my family:

Thank you, my amazing siblings, Jill (thank you for the book title), Diane, Richard, Lizzie, Anthony, and your families for your love and fabulous sense of humor. It's great to travel through life with your big hearts and laughs.

I am blessed with wonderful parents. Thank you to my mom, Sonnie, for all your care and love and for your sense of humor and zaniness that I am lucky enough to share. Big hugs and love.

To my dad, Ziggy, thank you for being my best cheerleader. Your guidance and support throughout my life helped me know anything is possible. Such a blessing! Love you!

To my stepmom, Lois, and my in-laws Enid, Al, Calvin, and Jane for surrounding our family with love and wisdom.

To our sons, Sam and Alexander, thank you for your kindness and wisdom. You challenge me, teach me, and bring me joy every single day. It's a gift to be your mom. I love you!

Finally, to my wonderful husband, Elliot. Your unwavering support, patience, guidance, eye for editing, and amazing cooking got me through this process! Thank you, Petey, for being my partner and traveling through life with me. Your love, I mean LOVE, means so much!

Live. Love. Laugh. Breathe.

LOVE & Gratitude,

Lauren

LAUREN CHELEC CAFRITZ is an internationally known breathwork coach, teacher, and speaker. As the founder of Experience Breath, she brings guidance, compassion, and joy to her clients in both individual and group breathwork sessions. She also lectures and facilitates breathwork sessions for nonprofits, government agencies, corporations, and schools and hosts retreats in sacred sites across the United States.

Through her experience as a businessperson, wife, mother, photojournalist, nonprofit advocate, and past sufferer of chronic pain, Lauren brings a unique perspective to her breathwork facilitation and nurtures her clients in a safe environment as they transform their lives. She is passionate about sharing the possibilities of healing and growth that come with breathwork.

Lauren has been featured in several national publications, radio shows, blogs, and podcasts. She is trained and certified in Integrative Breathwork and Transformational Breath® and has studied many other breathing modalities. Lauren serves as the United States representative for the International Breathwork Foundation and is a member of the Global Professional Breathwork Alliance.

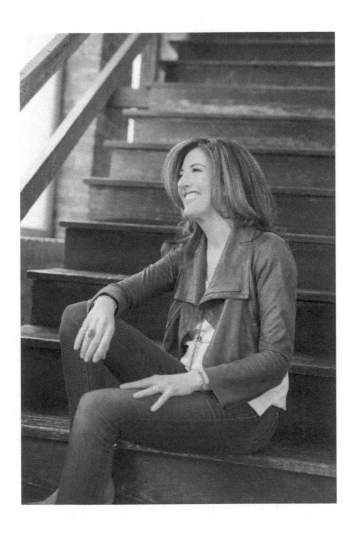

CPSIA information can be obtained
at www.ICGtesting.com
Printed in the USA
FFHW022200240719
53860829-59555FF